REPRODUCTIVE BEHAVIOUR AND HEALTH CARE PRACTICES

Haradhan Mandal

RAJAT PUBLICATIONS
New Delhi

Reproductive Behaviour and Health Care Practices
by *Haradhan Mandal*

This edition is published by Rajat Publications
4740/23, Ansari Road Daryaganj,
New Delhi - 110002

ISBN: 978-81-7880-235-0

Edition 2025
Rs. 1695/-

Printed and bound in India

RAJAT
PUBLICATIONS

4740/23, Ansari Road, Daryaganj,
New Delhi- 110002 (India)
Mob:- +91-9811484973, +91-9811105389
E-mail: rajat_publication@yahoo.com

ACKNOWLEDGEMENT

I place on record my deep sense of gratitude to my guide, Dr. Kashi Kailash Nath Sharma. He extended me a very able guidance and moral support. I am very much indebted to him.

I shall be failing in my duties if I do not express my sincere gratitude to Dr. Prof. Ramesh Chaube, Head, Deptt. of Anthropology, Dr. Harisingh Gour University for his valuable suggestions and constant inspiration in finalising this study.

I must acknowledge my indebtedness to my brother, friend and philosopher Dr. Dipak Kumar Adak, Research Associate Anthropological Survey of India, Sagar Field Station, Sagar, M.P. and my ex-student Dr. Niranjan Kumar Ghatak, Joint Director, Ministry of Tribal Affairs, Government of India, Shastri Bhavan, New Delhi, who extended me constant encouragement during this study. They have always been perennial source of inspiration for me.

I am grateful to Dr. Palash Coomar, Deputy Director, Census Operation, West Bengal for providing me necessary facilities for carrying out this study I am indebted to the Library Staff, Director of Census Operation, West Bengal. India Statistical Institute and Anthropological Survey of India, Kolkata for providing me library facilities.

I am thankful to Dr. P. Bharati, Dr. T.S. Vasulu, Dr. Bholanath Ghosh, Dr. Bechuram Mandal of Indian Statistical Institute, Kolkata. Sri Gautam Adhikary of Dept of Anthropology, Dinabandhu Mahavidyalaya, Bongaon. Sri Pradip Biswas, Sri Ajoy Biswas, Prof. Subalendu Mukhopadhyay, Sri Anup Chatterjee of Bongaon. Late

Sri Sanjay Kr. Yadav, Sri Ajay Kumar Gharami of Deptt. of Anthropology, Dr. Harisingh Gour University and a number of friends who have directly or indirectly helped me in various capacities.

I must thank to respondents of my field area who were very co-operative although the administration of various phases of data collections. I express my thanks to those authors whose work have been referred to my thesis.

I shall be failing in my duty if I do not acknowledge the help rendered by my wife Mrs. Dipa Mandal without whose sincere cooperation it would not have been possible to complete this empirical study within a short spell of time.

Thanks are due to Mrs. Seema Wasan and the associates of the Rajat Publications for the neat and prompt publication of this book.

Haradhan Mandal

CONTENTS

Acknowledgement *v*

1. Introduction 1

2. Area and the People 14

3. Material and Methods 36

4. Demographic characters 41

5. Reproductive Performance 73

6. Health Care Practices 101

7. Discussion and Conclusion 124

Bibliography 134

Index 156

1

INTRODUCTION

Indian society consists of numerous social, ethnic, linguistic, religious and territorial groups, which by and large reside in villages where poverty, illiteracy, ignorance and superstitions prevail. Indian rural economy is based predominantly on agriculture. Land is the basic means of production in rural economy. Land is a part of nature, though made arable by human labour. From land, the rural people produce, by means of technique and their labour power, such a variety of agrarian products as food, cotton, jute, tea, coffee, tobacco and others. But the main economic source, the land is generally owned by several middle and higher class and caste groups. The scheduled castes, scheduled tribes and other backward castes from the economically weaker sections in the society. Most of them live in the villages. In West Bengal, in general, and North Twenty Four Paraganas District in particular the scheduled castes group lead a precarious economic life and their health status too is generally very poor.

It is difficult to ascertain why people want more children as it is associated with economic, social and psychological considerations, which cannot be easily disentangled. The situation also varies from society to society and among individuals within a society. In many societies it is found that parents' reproductive goals, where they exist, are based on the number of children expected to survive them and care for them in their old age, they must have-in high- mortality country (ESCAP, 1988). Such a level of fertility is close to a biological ceiling for all practical purposes.

To-day the most urgent and important problem, which is standing before us and affects the well being of mankind, is the rapid growth of population.

India holds a special position in the world in terms of population. It is one of the oldest civilisations in the world. People have inhabited it for thousands of years. No wonders, at present it constitutes one of the most crowded parts in the world. According to 1991 census, India's population was 844 million, which had increased to 950 million by 1997. It is estimated that by 2005 India's population would be 1400 million, which is likely to increase further to 1800 million by 2075 (Chandna, 1999).

Growing population numbers have equally serious socio-economic implications at global, national and household levels. While at individual household level, social awakening through education may hold the key to the change in the perspective, at national and global levels thoughtful population planning policies, capable of producing both immediate and long term gains are needed (Chandna, 1999).

India's current demographic phase is characterised by rather high fertility and moderate mortality rates. As a result, the country's population is growing rapidly with about 18 million people being added to it annually, to give a 2.1 per cent increase per annum (Rao, 1996). In order to check the growth of population it is essential to understand the process through which the fertility behaviour is regulated in different cultural groups. The norms, values, customs and taboos prevalent in a society regulate reproductive behaviour. To understand the fertility behaviour of any group, these norms and values must be pinpointed.

Reproductive behaviour in animals includes all the events and actions that are directly involved in the process by which an organism generates at least one replacement of it self. In the evolutionary sense, the goal of an individual in reproduction is not to perpetuate the population or the species, rather, relative to the other members of its population, it is to maximise the representation of its own genetic characteristics in the next generation. The dominant form of reproductive behaviour for achieving this purpose is sexual (Encyclopaedia Britannica, 1983).

Reproductive behaviour of man was channalised by marriage, which is a vital, social as well as cultural institution in human society. In the Hindu society marriage is regarded as a necessity for the procreation of children. There is a Sanskrit saying "Putrarthe Kriate Varya" means one selects a wife only to have a son.

Reproductive patterns and behaviour- age at marriage, timing and spacing of birth, and family size—directly impinge upon the viability of young children and the probability of their survival (Ruzicka and Kane, 1987).

While adopting the constitution on January 26, 1950, we, the people of India, dedicated us to the creation of a new social order based on equality, freedom, justice and the dignity of the individual and, to that end, decided to eliminate poverty, ignorance and ill-health.

As defined in the constitution of the World Health Organisation (WHO) "health is a state of complete physical, mental and social well being and not merely the absence of disease or infirmity".

The health of a society is intimately related to its value system, its philosophical and cultural traditions and its social, economic and political organisation. Since each of these aspects has a deep influence on health and since health in its turn, also influences all these aspects, it is not possible to raise the health status of a people unless such efforts are integrated with the wider effort to bring about the overall cultural, social, economic and political transformation of the society as a whole. Such coordinated and simultaneous efforts to improve health status and change the entire social order generally yield better results because they are interdependent and mutually supportive. This is the entire more so if one is planning for the health of the people and not merely for health services. In fact, good health and good societies go together.

Health seeking is an important factor in health management,

but in a country like India, where most of the health schemes are centralised, this is often ignored while considering for providing health facilities to people. As a result, new schemes for providing health do not get the desired acceptance of the community and are therefore, rendered unsuccessful. The decision makers in the health are recognising the need for understanding the health seeking behaviour and perception of the communities and their acceptance and use of traditional and modern methods, as also the perception of the community regarding the service delivery. This is especially relevant to the communities of weaker section, where due to their under-exposure and strong beliefs in traditional culture, there is strong influence of age – old traditions and values (Singh, 1999).

The health status of population is determined not only by the availability and the level of health facilities but also by the ability to take advantage of these by various groups of the people. It is observed that public health centres are essentially curative, capital intensive and are oriented towards the rich and the urban areas. The fact remains that the urban areas generally get the lion's share of medical resources. While assessing their impact in rural areas it is necessary to throughly examine if the public health centres are well equipped in terms of professional expertise and staff members. However, the fact remains that though the public facilities are to play dominant role in the lives of the patients belonging of the rural areas, but their performances have not be perfect and adequate in many areas (Gupta, 1998).

World Bank in his February 1980's report in the report in the titled " Health – sector policy paper" states that the health problems of developing countries can be controlled or treated with presently known technologies. Infectious diseases could be reduced through good hygiene, early diagnosis and treatment and immunisation. Improvements in water supply and waste disposal would greatly facilitate control of fecal related diseases, but good personal hygiene, careful preparation of food, and use of safe drinking water are also essential. Immunisation against the most common and serious childhood diseases, such as measles polio, tetanus, diphtheria and pertusis are available at moderate cost. Use of better weaning foods and continuation of breast-feeding would reduce early childhood malnutrition and diminish the seriousness of infectious diseases. Parental care, screening for difficulties in delivery, safe delivery and neonatal care would drastically reduce maternal and neonatal mortality and greatly improve the health prospects of children.

Health care is a high priority in all developing countries and is a constitutional right in a number of them. The term primary health care is defined by a conference convened by WHO and UNICEF at Alma-Ata, USSR, in September 1978. It means, "essential health care based on practical, scientifically sound and socially acceptable methods, and technology made universally accessible to individuals and families in the community and country can afford......(It) addresses the main health problems in the community providing promotive, preventive, curative and rehabilitative services accordingly,..... (and) includes at least; education concerning prevailing health problems and the methods of preventing and controlling them; promotion of food supply and proper nutrition; and adequate supply of safe water and basic sanitation; maternal and child health care, including family planning; immunisation against the major infectious diseases; prevention and control of locally epidemic diseases; appropriate treatment of common diseases and injuries; and provision of essential drugs." The term basic health care refers to maternal and child health care, family planning, immunisation, prevention and control of epidemic diseases and treatment of common diseases and injuries, but excludes such health-related activities as education, nutrition, water supply and sanitation".

There is urgent need to update our present knowledge about health status and health care practices among the weaker section especially scheduled caste population.

In view of the above backdrop it is proposed to undertake an intensive study on reproductive behaviour and health care practices among the Namasudra, a scheduled caste of West Bengal with special reference to Bongaon Block in North Twenty Four Parganas.

Review of Literature:

The fertility behaviour is affected by biological factors and personal preference and indirectly by social customs and collective preferences. All these biosocial factors are therefore should be taken into account while formulating an effective population policy of a country (Sadhu, 1957).

Studies on menarcheal age and menopause with relation to fertility pattern have been conducted by several scholars (Seetha, 1957; Rakshit, 1962; Memoria, 1965: Bardhan, 1966; Biswas, 1967; Buck and Stavarky, 1967: Khan, 1973; Goyal, 1974; Rami Reddy, 1977 and Thomas, 1987). In another study Pandey and Tiwary (2000) estimated the vital rates of the primitive tribes of Madhya Pradesh.

Different scholars studied effects of age at first marriage, number of wives and types of marital union on fertility. Age at first marriage is one of the most important variables affecting fertility (Hajnal, 1963). Within marriage there is contradictory evidence on whether wives in polygynous union have lower completed fertility than those in monogamous unions (Smith and Kunz, 1976). It has also been suggested (Van de Walle, 1968; Page, 1975) that women in defacto unions tend to have lower fertility than women in formal marriages.

The influence of age at marriage on fertility is relatively minor under condition of natural fertility (Henry, 1976). Women who are married at a late age may practice shorter birth intervals therefore, catch up in child bearing with women who marry at an early age (Henry, 1961). Others reports equal fertility in polygamous and monogamous unions (Busia, 1954); Olusanya, 1971; Pool, 1968; Ohadike, 1968; Okore, 1977; Orubuloye, 1977). Yet others indicate higher monogamous than polygamous fertility (Muhsam, 1956; Brebant, 1954; Brito, 1952; Van - de Walle, 1968; Dorjahn, 1959; Stanley, 1956; Smith and Blacker, 1963).

Different scholars have studied family type with relation to fertility pattern. During the past 25 years many demographic studies have examined the relationships between family composition and fertility but their findings have been largely inconclusive. Lorimer (1954), Davis (1955) and Davis and Blake (1956) held that extended family systems support early marriage, which encourages high fertility and the nuclear families and later marriages are characterised by lower fertility. But several more recent Indian studies (Driver, 1963; Nag, 1967; Prakasi and Malaker, 1967; Bebarta, 1977; Mahadevan, 1979) have contradicted these theoretical expectations by reporting that joint families have lower fertility. This negative association has been explained by lack of privacy in joint households (Driver, 1963; Nag, 1967), taboos upon intercourse leading to lower coital frequency (Nag, 1967; Mahadevan, 1979). Still other studies have found little or no significant variation in fertility according to family type (Stycos, 1958; Freedman *et al.*, 1964; Palmore, 1972). Karim (1974) found that Pakistan women in joint families had a smaller average family size than those in nuclear families.

The increase in average age at marriage plays a positive role in reducing fertility as shown by various studies (Mukherjee, 1962; Barrai *et al.*, 1968; Bumpass, 1969; Matsunga and Tonomura, 1972; Selvin and Garfinkel, 1976; Mastunga, 1973; Goyal, 1975; Luella, 1974; Mo-Im *et al.*, 1974; Chouhan, 1974 and Dandekar, 1974). Pandey *et al.* (2001) conducted a study on the correlates of infant morality in a primitive tribe of Madhya Pradesh.

Poor environmental and sanitary conditions are associated with high infant and child mortality (Da Vanzo *et al.*, 1983; Trussell and Hammerslough, 1983; Jain, 1985; Merrick, 1985; Rahman, 1985; Victoria *et al.*, 1988; Gubhaju *et al.*, 191).

Diarrhoea is a major problem in developing countries and caused an estimated 2.9 million deaths in 1992 (Grant, 1994). At least a further three million children die annually in developing world from consequence of respiratory infections (Pio *et al.*, 1984; Leowski, 1986).

Control of food and water born diseases (diseases of dirty hands) in possible through promotion of personal hygiene (Stanton *et al.*, 1988; Henry and Rahim, 1990) in conjunction with improved water supply sanitation (Briscoe, 1987; Briscoe et al., 1988; Manun'ebo *et al.,* 1994) and sanitary disposal of faeces (Baltazar and Solon, 1989; Han and Moe, 1990). Lower socio-economic status, an unclean domestic environment, use of non- purified water, absence of soap and feeding methods other than exclusive breast feeding in early infancy are also risk factors for diarrhea (Huttly *et al.*, 1987).

Benefits of breast-feeding in protecting young infants against common childhood diseases such as diarrhea and respiratory diseases are well known (Mata and Wyatt, 1971; Chandra, 1978; Jelliffe and Jelliffe, 1978; Janowitz *et al.*, 1981). Breast-fed children experience considerably lower risk of morbidity and mortality than non – breast fed children (Robinson, 1951; Plank and Milanesi, 1973; Cunningham, 1983; Goldberg *et al.*, 1984; Adlakha and Suchindran, 1985).

Research based on data from diverse sources provides convincing evidence of positive effects of breast feeding and long birth intervals on infant survival (Cleland and Sathar, 1984; De – Sweemer, 1984; Forste, 1994; Hobcraft *et. al.*, 1985; Koenig *et al.*, 1990; Kuate Defo and Palloni, 1995; Lantz et al., 1992; Muhuri and Menken, 1997).

Increasing concern over infant and maternal health in developing countries has focussed new attention and its impact on health, nutrition and fertility (Buchanan, 1975). In addition, breast-feeding makes a major contribution to fertility control by lengthening the period of post-partum amenorrhoea (Perez *et al.*, 1972).

The level of educations of husband and wife and their economic status also play important role in child bearing age of mother (Nayer, 1974; Gupta *et al.*, 1975; Frisancho *et al.*, 1974; Chouhan, 1974). Education is a direct and powerful indicator of the status of women. However, the relationships between education and fertility are complex. It is intricately associated with many social, economic and psychological factors and attitudes. Education depresses fertility by raising the age at marriage, fostering a favourable attitudes towards small family size norm and improving awareness and use of family planning methods. A number of studies (Singh, 1989; Patnaik, 1985; Gomti Arora, 1990 and Vashisht *et al.*, 1991) have brought out clearly the impact of female education on reduction of fertility.

Population growth is the result of desire for more children and preference to male sex (Novitsky and Kimball, 1958; Pareek and Kothandapani, 1969; Raina, 1969; Gustavus and Nam, 1970; Culright *et al.*, 1974; Stinner and Madar, 1975; Talwar, 1965 and Coombs, 1979).

Fertility in relation to parity has been studied by Yerushalonyo (1945), Freedman and Coombs (1966), Grabill and Davidson (1968), James (1969), Bhanot and Gandotra (1970) and Khan (1973).

Nutrition, socio-economic condition and state of health effect the menarcheal age and menopause and in turn determine the reproductive span of women. This has been studied by various scholars (Clegg and Harrison, 1971; Baker and Dutta, 1972; and Dutta, 1980).

A number of surveys has been carried out on the incidence of consanguineous marriages and its influence on fertility and mortality (Dronamaraj and Meera Khan, 1963; Sanghvi, 1966, 1978; Basu, 1971, 1978 and 1986; Chakraborty, 1968; Kumar, 1967; Mukherjee and Bhaskar, 1974; Chakraborty and Chakraborty, 1973, 1977; Rao and Reddi, 1977; Goswami, 1970; Rao and Inbaraj, 1979 and Reddi, 1987; Mitra, 2000 and Pandey, 2002).

Health and disease are a continuous process and are linked to the health seeking behaviour of a community. A number of factors have been reported to influence the health seeking behaviour of individuals among which the socio – cultural pattern of the community is the most important (Rosenstock, 1960; Pandey and Tiwary, 1993).

Caldwell *et al.* (1983) points out that a child's mother is the person most likely to notice problem with a child's health because of her role as the primary carer, and she is therefore likely to be in the best position to make health care choices, but where women are likely to live in extended families with their mother-in-law, health care decision may often be made by the husband's mother or woman's mother-in-law rather than the woman herself.

As well as household decision-making processes, household resources are likely to influence the health and mortality of infant and children. Household production determines the capability of household to purchase health goods and services (Chatterjee, 1989; Doaen and Bisharat, 1990; Berman *et al.,* 1994; Berhrman, 1998). Basu (1987) found that a mother's ability to make her decision-making count was limited by the resources available to the household. It has also been argued that while the nuclear household may create more initiative to access health services, the joint household offers a better social security system for dependants and is therefore more likely to provide the necessary resources for seeking health treatment (Chakki, 1974; Caldwell *et al.*, 1996; Murthy *et al.*, 1985).

The effects of social, economic, occupational, educational and other cultural factors on fertility are generally known (Pearl, 1939; Lorimer *et al.,* 1954; UN, 1973; Nag, 1962; Bogue, 1969; Pandey, 2000) but while some studies reveal an inverse relationship between fertility and economic status (Whelpton and Kiser, 1950; US Bureau of the census, 1950; Chang, et al., 1979) others do not (US Bureau of the Census, 1953; Grabil *et. al.,* 1958; Bean and Wood, 1974). An inverse relationship between morality and economic status is also recognized and infant mortality is regarded by many as a measure of community health status (Yanakura, 1959). In the Indian context, such relationship of fertility and mortality with economic condition have been analysed recently by Mitra (1978), whereas Frisancho *et al.* (1976), show that low economic status is inversely related to fertility and childhood mortality.

The importance of cultural factors for fertility control in under developed countries has often been stressed (Chandrasekharan, 1959; Lorimer, 1954; Freedman, 1963; Opler, 1964; Schnaiberg, 1970; Khalifa, 1973; 1976). Yet few studies have actually attempted to measure their impact (cf, George , 1973). The measurement of traditionalism as such moreover, has generally been restricted to male subjects in developing countries (Larner, 1958; Smith and Inkeles, 1966; Kahl, 1968; Williamson, 1970; Poston and Singlemann, 1975). The exclusion of women, however, may be a serious shortcoming; indeed "a modern mother may be the central figure in bringing about societal modernisation" (Fawcett and Bornstein, 1973).

An important factor contributing to high fertility and low acceptance of family planning in less developed countries like India is high infant mortality (Chandrasekhar, 1972). It is particularly in these countries that control of fertility through promotion of family planning is an urgent issue, to prevent population growth.

Evidences from recent studies on the interrelation between mass media and family planning in developing countries support the claim that mass media do influence behaviour (Bertrand *et al.,* 1987; Piotrow *et al.,* 1990). Westoft and Rodriguez (1993) examine the relationship between exposure to media messages on family planning and a number of indicators of reproductive behaviour (including ever and current use of contraceptive, intention to use among non-users, desire for more children and ideal family size). The results indicate that women who are exposed to such messages in the media are more likely to use contraceptives and to desire fewer children. Evidence from a focus group study (Bankole, 1994) shows that this is indeed possible. Responses to the question on media exposure may be affected by selective recall. For instance, women have used or are currently using family planning methods may be more sensitive to media messages about family planning and may be more likely to report having heard or seen such messages than those who have not used any method (Westoff and Rodriguez, 1993).

Universal and prolonged breast-feeding in developing countries has the twin effects of lengthening birth intervals and reducing infant mortality (Jain and Bongaarts, 1981). The health benefits of breastfeeding have been discussed in detail (Mc Cann *et al.*, 1981; Van Landingham, *et al.,* 1991). Breast milk is a vital source of nutritious uncontaminated food for infants.

In the last decade, there has been a tremendous increase in the literature on fertility and family planning. Attempts have been made both in India (Dandekar, 1959; Mysore population study, 1961; Driver, 1963; Mamdani, 1972) and abroad (Hill *et al.*, 1959; Meier, 1959; Freedman, 1967) to develop theories or models on fertility and family planning behaviours. They have succeeded in pointing out some of the determinants of fertility behaviour, but still the picture of the whole mechanism which regulates fertility behaviour is not clear (Marshal, 1972; Sinding, 1974). Realising the scarcity of 'grand 'or even "middle range" theories on fertility and family planning, several scholars such as Bogue (1966), Fawcett (1970), Pohlman (1969), Youkey (1969) have emphasised the need for developing a model and conceptual frame-work for the analysis of fertility behaviour.

The health of mothers and their young children are closely

related, especially during gestation and in the neonatal period (Mubarak, 1989; Tinker and Koblinsky, 1993). It has been estimated that 99 percent of the world's maternal deaths and 50-60 percent of infant deaths in developing countries occur within one month of birth, mainly because of lack of maternal health care (Bolam *et al.*, 1998; World Health Organisation, 1996). The International Conference on Population and Development (ICPD) of 1994 focussed on reproductive health, with the objective of enabling women to go safely through pregnancy and childbirth and providing couples with the best chance of having a healthy infant. The ICPD policy document says that both mother and child have the right to appropriate health care services (United Nations, 1994).

Most studies of maternal and child health have focussed on social, economic, environmental and demographic patterns in infant and child mortality (Gubhaju, Streatfield and Mazumder, 1991; Gubhaju, 1985; Pant, 1996). Lack of antenatal care is also a major cause of neonatal mortality (Miller *et al.*, 1996; Clarke and Coward, 1991; Bhatia and Cleland, 1995; Foege, 1983). Several risk factors are closely associated with insufficient antenatal care, age of mother, education, birth order, poverty and geographical location (Wallace, 1992). If the mother is in good health and free of complications, she may be able to deliver at home safely (Poovan *et al.*, 1990; Drejer, 1991). On the other hand, some women who do not receive medical supervision during the pregnancy period may be at risk, but not recognised as being in high-risk category. So have delivery could pose dangers for both baby and mother.

It is hypothesized that the availability of health care infrastructure, personel and services has a positive impact on children's health outcomes, that access to health care has a greater effect among the poor than the non-poor, and that mothers with formal schooling use the health care system more efficiently to improve the health of their children than mothers with no formal schooling. An improved understanding of the causal relationship between the health services supply environment and health status, and the identification of which groups benefit most from the availability of government services, should be useful to government policy makers responsible for expanding health care and nutrition programmes in rural communities (Hotchkiss *et al.*, 2002).

The caste system is a unique feature of the Indian social structure and has a considerable influence on the individual's personality and life-style. In the study of any kind of social behaviour, it is desirable that caste should be taken as an independent variable and its influence is understood properly. It has been observed in several studies (Wyon and Gordon, 1971; Rele, 1963; Saksena, 1973) that higher caste couples had relatively lower fertility than those of low caste couples.

In national health policy scheduled caste groups become priority groups. A critical review of the literature clearly shows that there are only few valuable investigations have been made so far on fertility, mortality differentials among these guoups in India and hardly any anthropological study conducted ever in this on Namasudra scheduled caste population of West Bengal (Mukhopadhyay, 1981; Ghatak, 1990; Basu *et al.,* 1992 and Sarkar, 2000) which is an urgent need for meaningful policy to provide better health care services.

Keeping the above in view the present study has been carried out among the Namasudra scheduled caste population of North 24 Paraganas of West Bengal.

The Objectives of the Study

1. To study reproductive variables (i.e. menarcheal age, age at marriage, menopause) and their relationships with reproductive profiles;
2. To ascertain their fertility and mortality profiles and associated socio – cultural factors;
3. To study their concept of health, perception and treatment of diseases and performances of availed health care services and
4. To understand the extent of awareness and use of family planning methods and its impact on fertility behaviour.

2

AREA AND THE PEOPLE

The State of West Bengal occupies an area of 88752.0 km^2 (Census of India, 1991) which accounts only 2.70 percent of the total area of the Indian Union (3,287,782 km^2).

This state has been divided into eighteen districts and each district comprises a number of sub-divisions. There are total 54 sub-divisions. Each sub-division is again comprised of a number of police stations and community development blocks. There are 339 numbers of community development blocks in the state. The boundaries of the community development blocks have been delineated on the basis of the contiguous jurisdiction line number.

The state is characterised by diversified relief and drainage system ranging from lofty mountain to coastal plain. Physiographically the state has three main regions namely (1) mountain (2) plateau and (3) plain. The rivers originating from the Himalayas and Chotanagpur plateau have formed the drainage system in the state. The major river Ganga and its tributaries like Tista, Torsa, Mohananda, Jaldhaka, Raidak and Punarbhaba originating from the Himalayas and the river like Dwarka, Ajoy, Mayurakshi, Damodor, Silai, Kasai, Rupnarayan Dwarakeswar and Subarnarekha are flowing in the State.

The climate of West Bengal in general is tropical. The sub-

Himalayan or plains are hot except during the short winter season. The Himalayan or the mountainous region in the north is cold on account of its latitude. The annual rainfall of the Himalayan and Sub-Himalayan regions are 2,000 mm and 1,400 to 1,600 mm respectively. The mean monthly temperature ranges from 16°C in the month of December to a maximum of 33°C in May in sub-Himalayan region. The maximum and minimum temperature of the Himalayan region is below 24°C and below 5°C respectively. The state is characterised by four major types of forest namely tropical semi evergreen forest, tropical moist, deciduous forest, littoral and swamp forest and tropical dry deciduous forest.

North Twenty-Four Parganas District

The present investigation was carried out among Namasudra scheduled caste of Bongaon in North Twenty Four Parganas District of West Bengal, where they are largely concentrated. The following account gives general features of this district.

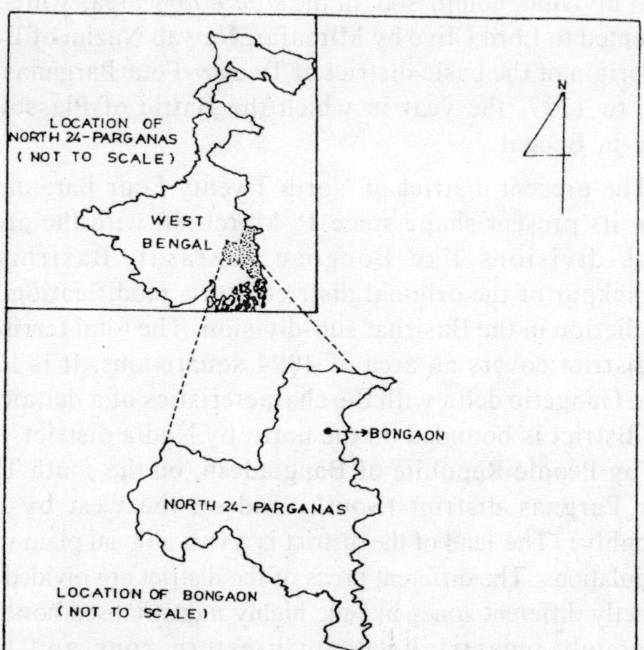

MAP 1: LOCATION OF NORTH 24-PARGANAS IN WEST BENGAL

The North Twenty-Four Parganas District is located on the south eastern part of West Bengal and it lies between 20°15'2" and 22°11'6" north latitude and 89°5' and 88°20' east longitude (Map 1).

Brief History of the District

The district of North Twenty-Four Parganas is included in the presidency division of the state of West Bengal from the year 1986 as per the Gazette Notification No. 212-LR/6MIS/83 dated 17-02-86. Before this notification this district was included in original district of Twenty-Four Parganas (24-Parganas). The present district has been formed with the northern areas of the undivided and unbroken Twenty Four Parganas District with Barasat as its administrative head quarter. The original district of Twenty-Four Parganas derives its name from the 24 numbers of Mahalas or Parganas, The fiscal division, comprised, in the *zamindary* areas which were presented to Lord Clive by Mirzafar, Nawab Nazim of Bengal. The origin of the basic district of Twenty-Four Parganas dated back to 1757, the year in which the Battle of Plassey took place in Bengal.

The present district of North Twenty Four Parganas has taken its present shape since 1st March'86 with the areas of 4 sub-divisions like Bongoan, Barasat, Basirhat and Barrackpur of the original district with a modification of the jurisdiction in the Basirhat sub-division. The total territory of the district covers an area of 4094 square kms. It is located in the Gangetic delta with the characteristics of a deltaic land. The district is bounded on the north by Nadia district, on the east by People Republic of Bangladesh, on the south Twenty Four Pargnas district (South) and on the west by Hugly (Hooghly). The land of the district is a vast alluvial plain without any dulations. The different areas of the district are divided into 3 distinctly different zones like the highly industrialised north zone; moderately industrialised north-estern zone and highly agricultural north-western zone. The main rivers of the district are Hugly, Ichamati, Jamuna and Kalindi.

The main source of livelihood of the people of the areas like Bongaon, Barasat and Basirhat sub-divisions is based on agriculture. And the persons of other sub-division are engaged in economic pursuit like industry, trade and other services. The major agricultural crops of the district are paddy, jute, oilseeds, pulses and vegetables. Metalled roads connect all the sub-divisional head quarters and all the police station headquarter's in the district. The different parts of the district are well served by arterial roads and railways.

History of Bongaon Sub-division

During 1880-81 Bongaon sub-division was included in the district of Nadia. In 1891, this sub-division was transferred from Nadia and included with the district of Jessore (At present it was included in Peoples Republic of Bangladesh). The district of Jessore was composed of five sub-divisions e.g. Jessore, Jhendia, Magura, Naral and Bongaon.

Population of Bongaon sub-division was 317352 in 1901 compared with 330,201 in 1891 (Census of India, 1981). It is a land of semi-stagnant rivers. The soil is comparatively poor, and the sub-division is more thinly populated (489 persons to the square miles) than the rest of the district. It contains one town Maheshpur (population 4,180) and 798 villages including Bangaon its headquarters. Under this sub-division there are four police stations or *thanas* like Mahespur, Sarsha, Bongaon and Gaighata.

By Notification No.549 G.A., dated 23rd February, 1948 the Bongaon sub-division was created with the police station Bongaon and Gaighata. The District consists of 6 sub-divisions like Sadar sub-division, Basirhat, Barasat, Bongaon, Barrackpur and Diamond Harbur (Map 2).

Bongaon Block

Bongaon block is located in North Twenty Four Parganas district

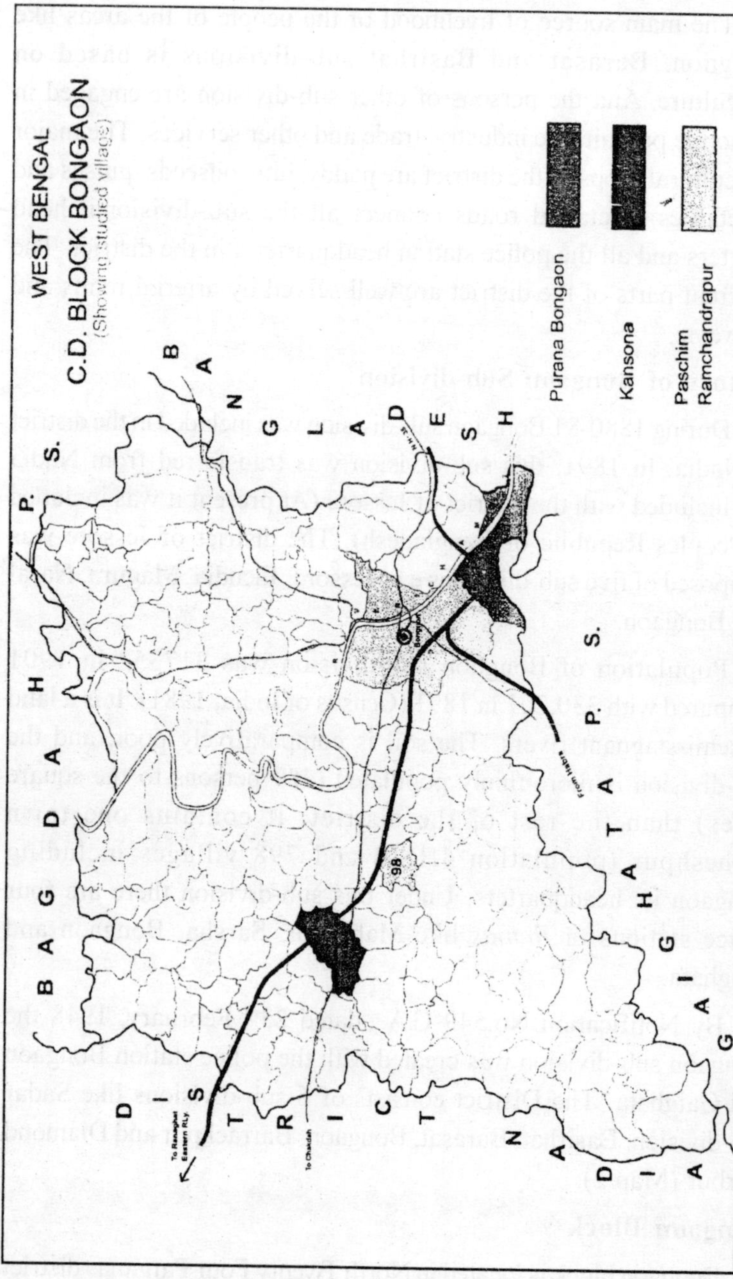
WEST BENGAL
C.D. BLOCK BONGAON
(Showing studied villages)
Purana Bongaon
Kansona
Paschim Ramchandrapur
From Habra
98

Bongaon block is located in North Twenty Four Parganas district of West Bengal, 77 km. from Kolkata. This block is situated by the western side of river Ichamati. The block Bongaon consists of 149 inhabited villages covering an area of 336.70 sq. kms. (Census of India, 1981). Main crops grown in this block are rice (aus, aman and boro varieties), wheat, barley, maize, potatoes, sugarcane, jute, pulses, mustered seeds. There are large numbers of big tanks (Baor is the local term) in this block and in such place sweet water fishes are cultivated in commercial basis. The important vegetations noted in this area are Teak (Tectona grandis), Pipal (Gicus religiosa), Siris (Albizzia lebbeck), Coconut (Cocos nuicfera), Indigo (Indigorera tinctoria), Neem (Azadiraehta tudiea), Babul (Acacia arabica), Bamboo (Bambusa tulda), Eucalyptus (Eucalyptus globosus), Jack fruit (Artocarpus integrifolia), Date palm (Phoenix sylvestris), Mast tree (Polyalthia longifolia), Mahogony (Swietenea maghogini) etc.

Historically this area is famous for three reasons. First of all famous historian and Indus valley civilisation excavator Sri Rakhaldas Bandyapadhya was born in Chhoyghoria. Secondly famous Bangali Novelist Sri Bibhutibhusan Bandhyapodhya was born in Barrackpur village and thirdly famous Bengali Dramatist Sri Dinabandhu Mitra (Nildarpan famous) was born in Chouberia.

According to 1981 census the total population of the Block was 229027 (118083 males and 110944 females). The population density per sq km is 680 and percentage of block population to district population is 4.14. According to 1991 census the total population of the block is 294432 (152479 are males and 141953 are females). Distribution of scheduled castes and scheduled tribes population of Bongaon block in the district North 24 Parganas is shown in Table 2.1.

Literacy (in percentage) of Bongaon Block in the district of North 24 Parganas is shown below according to 1981 and 1991 Census (Table 2.2).

Table 2.1

Scheduled Caste and Scheduled Tribe Population of Bongaon Block

Name of the Block	*Year (Census)*	*Scheduled Castes*			*Scheduled Tribes*		
		Males	*Females*	*Total*	*Males*	*Females*	*Total*
Bongaon	1981	52039	48699	100738	3719	3629	7348
	1991	71709	66646	138355	4819	4627	9446

Table 2.2

Per cent of litracy in Bongaon Block

Name of the Block	*1981 Census*			*1991Census*		
	Males	*Females*	*Total*	*Males*	*Females*	*Total*
Bongaon	44.2%	26.1%	35.3%	61.92%	42.85%	52.76%

Out of total 68,077,965 populations (According to 1991 Census) in the state the scheduled caste population has been noted to be 16,080,611 and it accounts 23.62 percent of total population. Among the different scheduled castes communities in the states, Rajbanshi are found as the most predominant community. Namasudra, the second largest scheduled caste, is mostly concentrated in Nadia, North Twenty Four Parganas and Jalpaiguri Districts.

The Namasudra

There are no documentary evidences about the origin of Namasudra. Manu brands them as "the lowest of mankind sprung from the illicit intercourse of a Sudra man with a Brahmin woman. In the Mahabharata they are introduced as hired assassins whose humanity however, revolt against putting an innocent boy to death. In the Ramayana they are described as ill formed and terrible in aspect, dressing in blue or yellow garments with a red cloth over the shoulders, a bear's skin around the Ioins and iron ornaments on the wrists. However, they are considered as a non-Aryan caste of Eastern Bengal, engaged for the most part in boating and cultivation. The derivation of this name is also uncertain. Dr. Wise thinks it may be from "the Sanskrit Namas adoration, which is always used as a vocative when praying or the Bengali Namate below underneath ". The letter suggestion seems the more plausible. The Pundits' interpretation of the former is understood to be that the Chandals is bound to do obeisance even to a Sudra. It would be promotion for the Chandals of Manu to get them recognised as a lower grade of Sudras. The name may also be referred to Namasa or Lomasa Muni; whom some Chandals regarded their mythical ancestor. On the other hand Namasa Muni himself may have been evolved from the attempt to explain always the suggestion of inferiority implied in the name Namasudra. (Risley, 1891).

The Chandals of Bengal invariably called themselves *Namasudra*, and with the characteristic jealously the higher division of the caste applies to the name Chandal to the lower, who in their term pass it on to the Dom. (Risley, 1981). They are regarded as untouchables by the higher caste of Bengal and only a generation ago was known by the name of Chandals. No doubt they are a somewhat backward community with a rather low level of culture who cannot point to any intellectual eminence or historical distinction among their forefathers in the immediate or distant past. But they are justified in rejecting the name of Chandal for their community as the Chandal of Dharmasutras was men who lived outside the pole of civilisation and settled life, and found maintenance from the most despised occupations.

The titles of the Namasudra are numerous. They are identified by the following title—Bagh, Bhala, Biswas, Das, Dhali, Dule, Hail, Halder, Hathi, Laskar, Mazumdar, Mandal, Mirdah, Mistri, Pradhan, Pandits, Paramanik, Patra, Rai, Santra, Singh etc.

The promotion of the Namasudras from the status of Chandals to that of second-class sudras is quite natural and is the consequence of the improved culture and way of living they have adopted. It was with the object of emphasising the fact that they were no longer Chandals that they adopted the name ending of Sudra, though they were ordinarily called *Namas*. As regards the claims of the Namasudras that they had formerly been Brahmans were degraded because they struck to Buddhism larger than other castes and who were given the name of sudra by the jealous Kayasthas, they are not supported either by history or tradition or anthropometry (Dutta, 1986).

Occupation

Previous records show that Namasudras are not occupational caste. Previously they were engaged in various persuits such as agriculture, navigating boats, carpentery, fishing etc. At present they are engaged in various occupations. During investigation in three villages the scholar came to know the different occupation like cultivation, agricultural labour, day labour, biri binding, hawkery, carpentry, drivery, teachers, services in government and private enterprise, chandsi doctor, business of rice making, tailor, rickshaw / van, puller, etc. were taken by the Namasudra. But Bose (1985) mentioned that besides agriculture navigating boats is also a traditional occupation of the Namasudra.

Habitation

Among three studied village (i.e., Purana Bangaon, Paschim Ramchandrapur and Kansona) most of the houses of Purana Bangaon and Paschim Ramchandrapur villages are kachha, i.e., wall is made by splitted bamboo and the roof is thatched by tiles, tin and hogla grass. The floor is made by bitted earth above the level ground. Each room is provided with a door made by tin or wood on a wooden frame. Some pacca houses made by brick wall and thatched roof is made by tin or tiles. On the other hand most of the houses in Kansona village are made by tin wall and tin roof. Most of the families have no pucca latrine.

Food and Drinks

Boiled rice is the staple diet of Namasudra. They usually take three meals a day and very few can afford a fourth. In the morning they take boiled rice soaked in water overnight with a pinch of salt, green chilies, onion and boiled potato. At noon they take boiled hot rice with pulses, vegetables and fish/ meat/ eggs. At night they also take rice with vegetable. Few of them take handmade breads with vegetables at night.

Presently tea is the popular drink of Namasudra. Almost in all families in the villages tea is taken in the morning and in the evening. The children drink cow-milk. They take tobacco in the form of smoking. Biri is the popular smoking cigarettes are also taken. Some of them rub the "gudaku" in their gums.

Dress and Ornaments

Ordinarily the Namasudra males wear *dhotis* and shirts. At present the adult males wear pant, shirt, *paijama* etc. The women use *sharies*, petticoats, and blouses, bra etc. The Namasudra woman use a variety of ornaments made by silver, golden and beads. The commonest ornament is a necklace made of silver and rarely of gold. They also like very much necklace of beads and city gold (chipper alloy metal) different kinds of earrings, finger rings etc.

Social Structure

The Namasudra are devided into a number of exogamaus groups based on occupation such as seuli, kora, kishore, nolo, mechho, nuniya and chasi.

Gotra

They have two gotras namely Kashyapa and Siva. They believed that the members of a particular gotra descended from certain saints or god. The members of Kashyapa gotra believed that they have descended from the saint Kashyapa and the members of Siva gotra also believed that their ancestor was Siva or Mohadev, the god of Kailash. The gotra is exogamous in nature.

Family

Majority of the Namasudra have nuclear family consists of a man, his wife, their unmarried children and father and mother. Some joint or extended families are also found among them. The families are patrilocal *i.e.* a girl after marriage goes to reside with her husband either in her husband's father family or in the individual family set up by her husband. At present some neolocal residence is also found. In the family the authority rests on the father but after the death of father the eldest son takes the position.

Marriage

Monogamy is strictly followed. Some sporadic cases of polygamy are prevalent among them. For marriage negotiation is the primary means of acquiring mates. Marriage by love is also found among them. Dowry is also found. Dowry is paid both in cash or kind. Divorce and re-marriage are allowed. In case of wife dies the husband is allowed to marry the wife's younger sister *(sororate).* Marriage rituals such as blessing the bride and bridegroom by elderly persons *(ashirbad),* smearing of turmeric paste on the bride and grooms *(gaye halud),* obtaining blessings from the ancestors, giving the daughter in marriage *(sampradan)* and servicing the rice for the first time by newly married bride *(boubhat)* are observed.

Inheritance and Succession

All the sons inherit parental property and at present the daughters also inherit the parental property.

Death and Funeral

The Namasudra usually cremate the dead body except in case of child. The dead child is buried. The dead body is cremated in a certain place known as *Sashan* (cremation ground) carried by relatives and friends and co-villagers on a wooden bier. After placing the dead body on a funeral pyre, the eldest son or near relatives puts a piece of burning wood in the face of the corpse. The mouring period lasts for ten days from the date of death. On the tenth day after death the head hair, beard and moustache of the mourner is shaved and the nail of hands and feet also cut down by the barber. The *shradhya* ceremony is held on 11th day and the rice and fish *(matshyamukhi)* feeding of the ceremonial party is held on the 13th day.

Religion

The Namasudras are Hindus and their family deities are Bhagabati, Bipadtarini, and Lakshmi etc. They observe Bastu-Puja, Pous Sankranti, and Dhane Sad Sitala, Manasa (goddess of snake), Basanti, Siva, Saraswati (goddess of learning), Durga and Kali are their regional as well as village deities. Charak and Durga Puja are the major festivals that are celebrated. At present most of them are followers of "Mothua religion" innovated by Sri Sri Harichand Thakur, a religious leader from the community of Orakandi, in Gopalganj district of present day Banladesh. He was born in 1812. He becomes active at a time when the untouchables of Bengal (undivided) were accepting Islam and Christianity due to illtreatment by the upper caste Hindus. He was addressed as an avatar of Bishnu. Lord' Harichand saved the untouchables from conversion by innovating Mothua Religion. His son Guruchand Thakur preached this religion among the Dalits and promoted their upward mobility by launching his famous education movement in 1881, 10 years

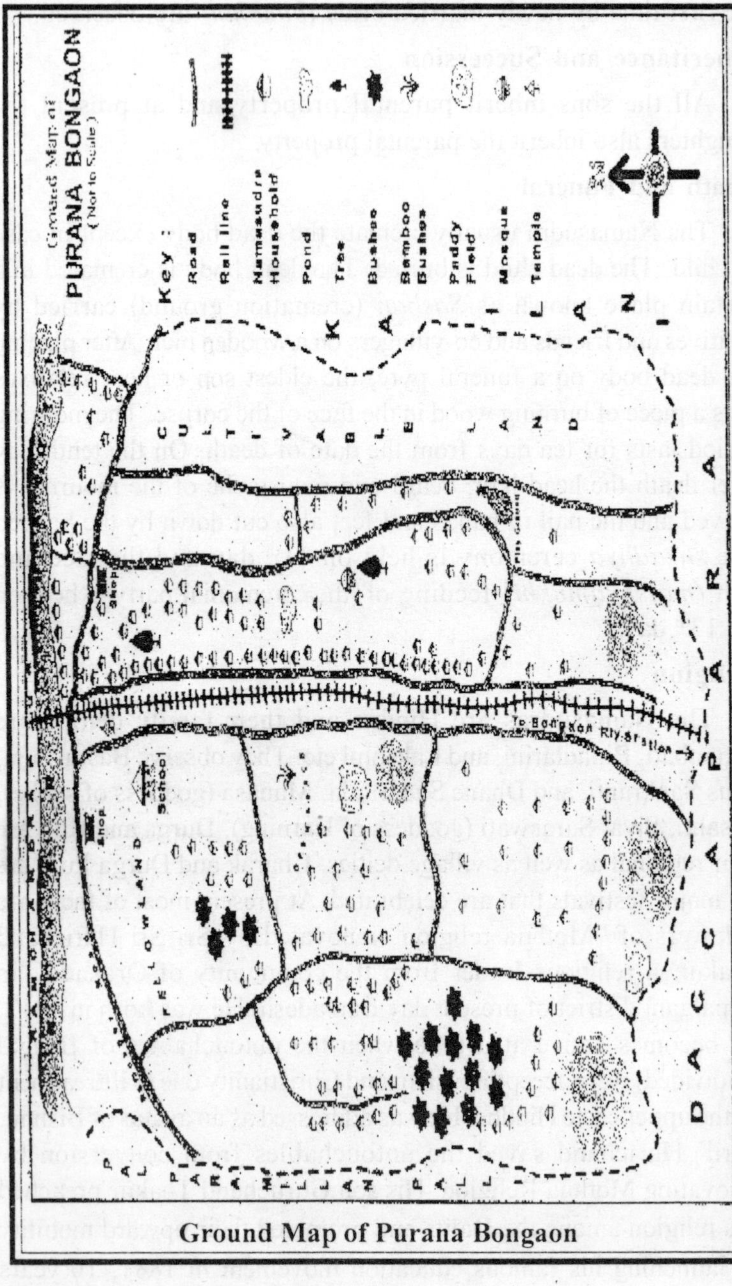

Ground Map of Purana Bongaon

before the birth of Dr. B.R. Ambedkar. Guruchand Thakur integrated Bengal's great Namasudra community into one unit from its eight divisions and skillfully organized their ongoing mass conversion to Motuaism in protest against Brahmanism (Walker, 2000). Every members of Mothuadharma worship god Hari. It is said that Sri Sri Harichand Thakur appeared in this community to keep the promise of Sri Chaitannya Deva at Nilachal (Orissa). The followers of this religious ideology are called themselves *Mothua*. The word Mothua has originated from the sense of being overjoyed with devotion for Hari, alias the Hindu god Sri Vishnu. They uttered the word Haribol.

A brief description of the three studied villages namely Purana Bongaon, Paschim Ramchandrapur and Kansona is given below:

Purana Bongaon

Purana Bongaon is situated at a distance of 3 km from Bongaon town and Sub-divisional Hospital (Dr. Jiban Ratan Dhar Sub-divisional Hospital). The north of Purana Bongaon is bounded by Ramchandrapur and it is separated by river Ichamati. The village Kailani is found to the east of Purana Bongaon. Dhakapara is found to the south and in west Palpara Milon Pally village is situated (Map 3). It is the main village within the gram panchyet of Kalupur. A pacca road connects Berigopalpur with Bongaon town via Purana Bongaon and only one bus route runs from Bongaon New market (Shyambazar Bus stand of Bongaon) bus stand to Berigopalpur via this village. The nearest railway station is at Bongaon Junction (Eastern Railway). It is partly electrified village. Previously no telephone and telegraph facilities do not exist. At present one telephone booth is installed in front of Sat Bhai Kalitala area from where S.T.D. and I.S.D. facilities are available.

Table 2.3

The Distribution of household and Population of village Purana Bongaon (as enumerated in December, 2000)

Serial No.	Community	Caste/SC/ST/ Other OBC	Total no. of households	Percents of household	Total Population
1.	Brahmin	General Caste	25	2.71	138 (3.06)
2.	Kayastha	General Caste	52	5.63	368 (8.17)
3.	Mahishya	General Caste	35	3.79	345 (7.66)
4.	Namasudra	Scheduled Caste	209	22.62	904 (22.06)
5.	Muslim	Minority Group	425	45.99	1863 (41.43)
6.	Kaibattra	Scheuled Caste	118	12.77	578 (12.83)
7.	Teli	Other Backward Caste	32	3.46	1.72 (3.06)
8.	Kamar	Other Backward Caste	28	3.03	138 (3.06)
	Total		**924**	**100.00**	**4506 (100.00)**

(Figures in parenthesis indicate percentage values)

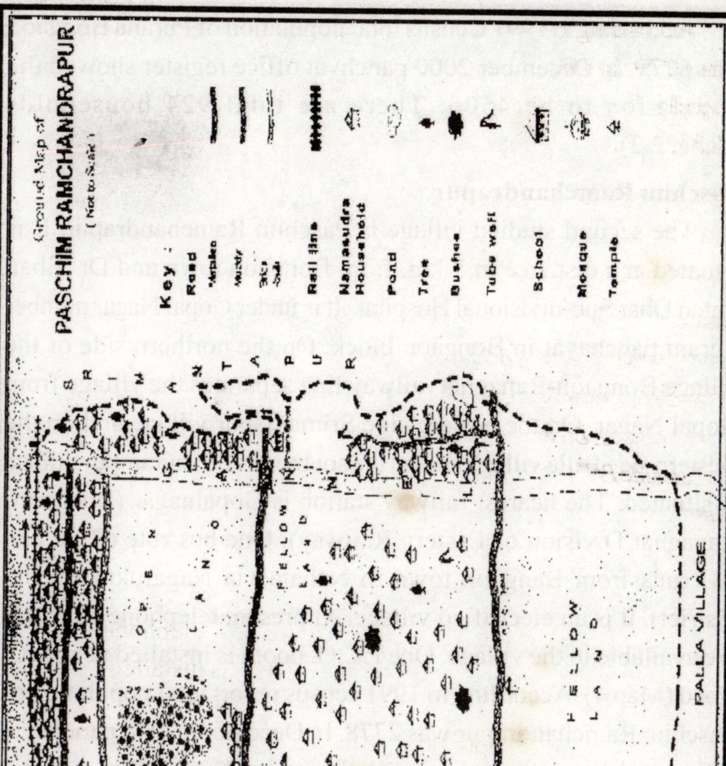

Ground Map of Paschim Ramchandrapur

According to 1991 Census total population of Purana Bongaon was 6279. In December 2000 panchyat office register showed the population to be 4506. There are total 924 households (Table 2.3).

Paschim Ramchandrapur

The second studied village is Paschim Ramchandrapur. It is situated at a distance of 7 km. from Bongaon town and Dr. Jiban Ratan Dhar Sub-divisional Hospital. It is under Gopal Nagar number I gram panchayat in Bongaon block. On the northern side of the village Bongaon-Ranaghat railway line separates the village from Gopal Nagar. On the eastern side Srimantapur village and on the western side Palla village and on the southern side Bairampur village is situated. The nearest railway station is Gopalnagar (Bongaon-Ranaghat Division of Eastern Railway). One bus rute (Rute No. 28) runs from Bangaon town to Nahata via Nagarukra (Nadia district). It is an electrified village. At present telephone facilities are available in the village. One P.C.O. booth is installed near N.C. Road (Map 4). According to 1991 census report total population of Paschim Ramchandrapur was 2778. In December, 2000 panchayat office register showed the population to be 3239. There are total 606 households (Table 2.4).

Kansona

The third studied village is Kansona. It is situated in Western side of Chakdah-Bongaon Road approximate 12 km. from Bongaon town and Dr Jiban Dhar Sub-divisional hospital. The main road connecting Bongaon and Chakdah (Bongaon-Chakdah Road) runs through the Kansona village. It bifurcates the village into two i.e., northern and southern. The village is included under Bairampur gram panchayat. The village is surrounded by Meherpur village in the north, Bairampur village in the south, Bardhamberia village in the east and Golakat in the west. It is fully electrified village. A branch post office has been set up in this village. Recently telephone

Table 2.4

The distribution of household and population of village Paschim Ramchandrapur (as enumerated in December, 2000)

Serial No	*Community*	*Caste/SC/ST/ Other OBC*	*Total no. of households*	*Percents of household*	*Total Population*
1.	Brahmin	General Caste	28	4.62	146 (4.50)
2.	Kayastha	General Caste	20	3.30	148 (4.56)
3.	Muslims	Minority Group	45	7.43	295 (9.11)
4.	Mahishya	General Caste	38	6.27	180 (5.56)
5.	Namasudra	Scheduled Caste	395	65.18	2023 (62.46)
6.	Napi	Other Backward Caste	5	0.42	28 (0.33)
7.	Muslim	Minority Group	438	36.59	3969 (47.33)
8.	Goala	Other Backward Caste	15	1.25	45 (0.45)
9.	Santal	Scheduled Tribe	188	15.70	809 (9.64)
	Total		**1197**	**100.00**	**8385** (99.99)

(Figures in parenthesis indicate percentage values)

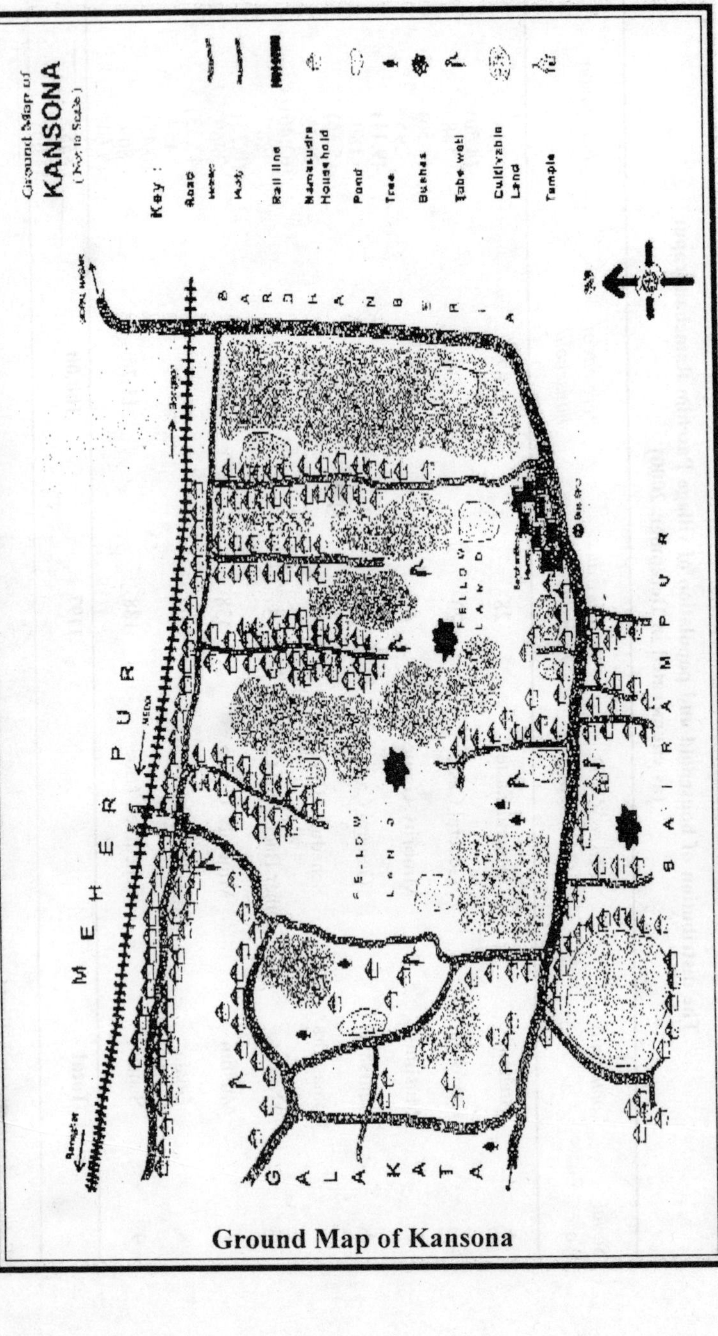

Ground Map of Kansona

Table 2.5

The distribution of household and population of village Kansona (as enumerated in December, 2000)

Serial No.	*Community*	*Caste/SC/ST/ Other OBC*	*Total no. of households*	*Percents of household*	*Total Population*
1.	Aliman	General Caste	157	13.12	8.72 (10.40)
2.	Bagdi	Scheduled Caste	85	7.10	402 (4.80)
3.	Bhaktadas	Other Backward Caste	82	6.85	1050 (12.52)
4.	Brahmin	General Caste	8	0.67	29 (0.35)
5.	Namasudra	Scheduled Caste	219	18.29	11.81 (14.08)

Cont...

Cont...

Serial No.	Community	Caste/SC/ST/ Other OBC	Total no. of households	Percents of household	Total Population
6.	Napi	Other Backward Caste	5	0.42	28 (0.33)
7.	Muslim	Minority Group	438	36.59	3969 (47.33)
8.	Goala	Other Backward Caste	15	1.25	45 (0.45)
9.	Santal	Scheduled Tribe	188	15.70	809 (9.64)
	Total		**1197**	**100.00**	**8385** (99.99)

(Figures in parenthesis indicate percentage values)

facilities are available in this village (Map 5). The nearest railway station is Gopalnagar and few government and private buses run from Bongaon town to Chakdah through Kansona. According to 1991 Census report, total population of Kansona was 6393. In December, 2000 panchayat office register showed the total population of to be 8385 comprising 1197 households (Table 2.5).

3

MATERIAL AND METHODS

Study Area

The present study has been carried out in North Twenty Four Parganas District of West Bengal.

Sampling

Bongaon block is purposively selected which have predominated concentration of Namasudra population compared to other blocks of the same district, to ensure maximum coverage of Namasudra community and to minimise the cost and time involved in the survey and to facilitate maximum utilisation of the time available for research.

The data of the present study were collected from three villages namely Purana Bongaon (Sat Bhai Kalitala), Paschim Ramchandrapur and Kansona on the basis of their locations from the Sub-Divisional Health Centre, situated in Bongaon town. These are as follows:

Village I – Purana Bongaon – located nearer to the Sub Divisional Health Centre (i.e. 3 km. far);

Village II – Paschim Ramchandrapur – located far from the Sub-Divisional Health Centre (i.e. 7 km. far) and

Village III –Kansona – located at a location furthest from the Health Centre (i.e. 12 km. far).

Sample Size

After grouping the villages into three categories, the three villages were selected using simple random technique from each group of villages. This was done on the basis of maximum concentration of the study population in the villages. Village Purana Bongaon is 3 km. away from Bongaon town, while distances of Paschim Ramchandrapur and Kansona from this town are 7 km. and 12 km. respectively. Information has been obtained from 876 ever married women. Out of which 202 from Purana Bongaon; 426 from Paschim Ramchandrapur and 248 from Kansona have been identified for in-depth interview.

Methods Applied for Data Collection

(i) Reproductive Variables, Fertility and Mortality Profile

Such data were collected from the households by interviewing the mothers with the help of structured schedules. Information on fertility and mortality were collected through pregnancy enumeration drawing genealogy with suitable crosschecks.

(ii) Attitude Towards Family Planning Methods

Data pertaining to this aspect were collected through case study methods. Side by side associated various socio-cultural factors were also studied.

(iii) Utilisation of Health Care Services

Information on concept of health, perception of disease, treatment of diseases, available facilities, utilisation and attitude toward modern health care services were colleted with the help of sehedule/questionnaire from selected households. Traditional village medicine men were also interviewed.

Before starting this study a pilot survey was undertaken in the study area in July 1999. The pilot survey was completed in February 2000.

Rapport Establishment

To begin with, the investigator moved around the study area and made friends with those who showed interest in him. The investigator then explained to them the purpose of his visits and used such friendships to extend the chain. The investigator meets the individuals of different age groups of the community and started communicating to them various problems and difficulties thus providing him opportunities to go deep into his data collection.

Besides this kind of group rapport, individual rapport was also very important. Having gained the confidence of the different strata and groups at large the investigator was able to come closer to these individuals, which helped the investigator for collection of various data.

After setting down in the study area and establishing rapport with the people there, the general sequence of work of investigator consisted in getting data concerning the physical features of the area, including the drawing of map, a general house to house survey of the village, interview for information, making direct observation of health behaviour of the Namasudra.

Members of the village Panchayat, Panchayat Samiti, School Teachers, Personel of the PHC hospital, social workers were among those who were interviewed relative to this study.

Besides using structured interview schedule, observation method was also employed for data collection. Though the collection of most of the information was obtained from the wife; data on certain items like age, education, marriage etc., were obtained from their husbands as they could provide relatively more reliable data.

During subsequent household visits, the wife and husbands were separately interviewed and data relating to delicate matter like elopment, abortion, contraception, use of herbal and ethno medicine by and taking amulet and for abortion or delay of conception were obtained. Beside these local *Dai, Anganwari* workers, health workers were also interviewed. All information colleted from three studied villages were continuously checked and households were visited repeatedly in order to increase the quality of information.

For the sake of analysis on economic status of the studied population three categories were made viz., (i) **high:** those mothers who belong to the families of high income group (per capita annual income more than Rs. 5000/=), (ii) **medium:** those mothers who belong to the families of medium income group (per capita annual income between Rs. 5000/= and 1001/=) and (iii) **low:** those mothers who belong to the families of low income group (per capita annual income Rs. 1000/= and less).

It may be mentioned that the investigator experienced great difficulties in assessing the age, particularly of the elderly women, since they were not aware of their real age. In these cases, we had to estimate their age with reference to some important local events and to the age of some other individuals, who seemed to be in the same age group. However, the age of the individuals are correct upto the month of birth, but not upto the date of birth.

Statistical Consideration

In order to interpret the data adequately the following statistical measures are incorporated.

A. Mean: Mean is the central value of a distribution. It is calculated by the following formula.

Mean : $\bar{x} = \sum x / n$,

Where $\bar{x}$ = mean value.

$\sum x$ = total of all values and

n = total number of observation.

B. Standard Deviation (S.D.) : Standard deviation is a measure of the extent to which the individual items vary. It is calculated by the following formula.

Standard Deviation (S.D.) : $\delta = \sqrt{\sum(x - \bar{x})^2 / n}$

Where $\bar{x}$ is the mean, 'x' is the individual observation and 'n' is the total number of observation.

C. Test of Significance :

I. **Chi-square (χ^2) test :** This test of significance is found useful in computing the difference in regard to non-metric data. It is defined as:

$\chi^2 = (O-E)^2 / E$,

Where O = observed frequencies and

E = expected frequencies.

For inference 0.05 probability level is taken into consideration in case of this test.

II. T – test : For the purpose of comparison among the various divisions the 't' – test of significance have been applied. This test is usually found convenient in examining the metric data.

Formula used for t-test is :

$t = M_1 - M_2 / \sqrt{d_1^2 + d_2^2}$

Where M_1 and M_2 stand for mean values of the two samples and d_1 and d_2 stand for the standard error of the two mean values respectively.

For inference 0.05 probability level is taken into consideration in case of this test.

D. Binomial test of equality of proportion :

This formula used as:

Sample size	Proportion	
N_1	n_1	$P_1 = n_1 / N_1$
N_2	n_2	$P_2 = n_2 / N_2$

$T_1 = P_1 - P_2$

$P = P_1 N_1 + P_2 N_2 / N_1 + N_2$

$q = 1 - p$

$T_2 = \sqrt{pq}\ \{(N_1 + N_2) / N_1 N_2\}$

If the T_1 is greater than twice T_2 ten the difference is significant.

4

DEMOGRAPHIC CHARACTERS

To the demographers the study of population composition constitutes a basic and the most relevant field of study. The composition of population is the internal structure of a human population with respect to one or more demographic attributes or traits at a particular point of time. The word 'composition' in population literature is often used as a synonym of 'distribution' or 'structure' (Misra, 1982). This varies in time and space as a consequence of birth as well as selective migration (Reddy, 1991). The study of population's composition, however, acts as an indicator of its current population dynamics (Chachra and Bhasin, 1998).

For the present study a door-to-door survey was conducted in three Namasudra villages namely Purana Bongaon, Paschim Ramchandrapur and Kansona. Age and sex distribution of the study population are shown in Tables 4.1, 4.1a, 4.1b and 4.1c respectively.

Age and Sex Structure

Distribution of the Namasudra population according to age and sex is shown in Table 4.1. Males are found to be more in number than the females when the total population according to age and sex is taken into consideration. Number of individuals gradually increases with the advancement of age from 0-4 years to 10-14 years in both the sexes. From 15-19 years onward however, a reverse trend is perceptible in the males and females both. Of the total population 31.02 per cent males and 34.30 per cent females fall in the group 0-14 years. While in 15-49 years age group 56.01 per cent males and 52.92 per cent females are found. The rest of the population fall in 50 years and above age group. The population pyramid (Fig. 4.1) shows a trend of progressive type population growth among the Namasudra.

In the preceding paragraphs distribution of the Namasudra population according to age and sex is described for the three villages separately.

In table 4.1a distribution of the Namasudra is set out for Purana Bongaon and in figure 4.2 the same has been presented graphically in the form of population pyramid. Of the total population, a significant excess of males relative to females is observed in this village. The number of total males is 478, whereas the number of total females is 426. It reveals that as the age increases the number of individuals gradually decreases in both the sexes. Of the total population 34.1 per cent males and 34.74 percent females fall in the age group 0-14 years, while in 15-49 years age group 54.39 per cent males and 53.29 per cent females are recorded. The rest of the population fall in 50+ year's age group. However, higher number of individuals is seen among the females than that of the males in 20-24 years and 25-29 years age group. But in 40-44 years age group a reverse trend is true. The population pyramid (Fig. 4.2 suggests a trend of progressive type population growth in this village.

In Table 4.1b the distribution of Namasudra population according to age and sex is set out for Paschim Ramchandrapur village and in figure 4.3 the same has been presented graphically in the form of population pyramid. Like the earlier village (i.e. Purana Bongaon) in this village also a significant excess of males (51.95 %) relative to females (48.05 %) is observed. There is a considerable increase of individuals from 0-4 years to 5-9 years age group in both the sexes. As the age increases the number of individuals gradually decreases in both the sexes.

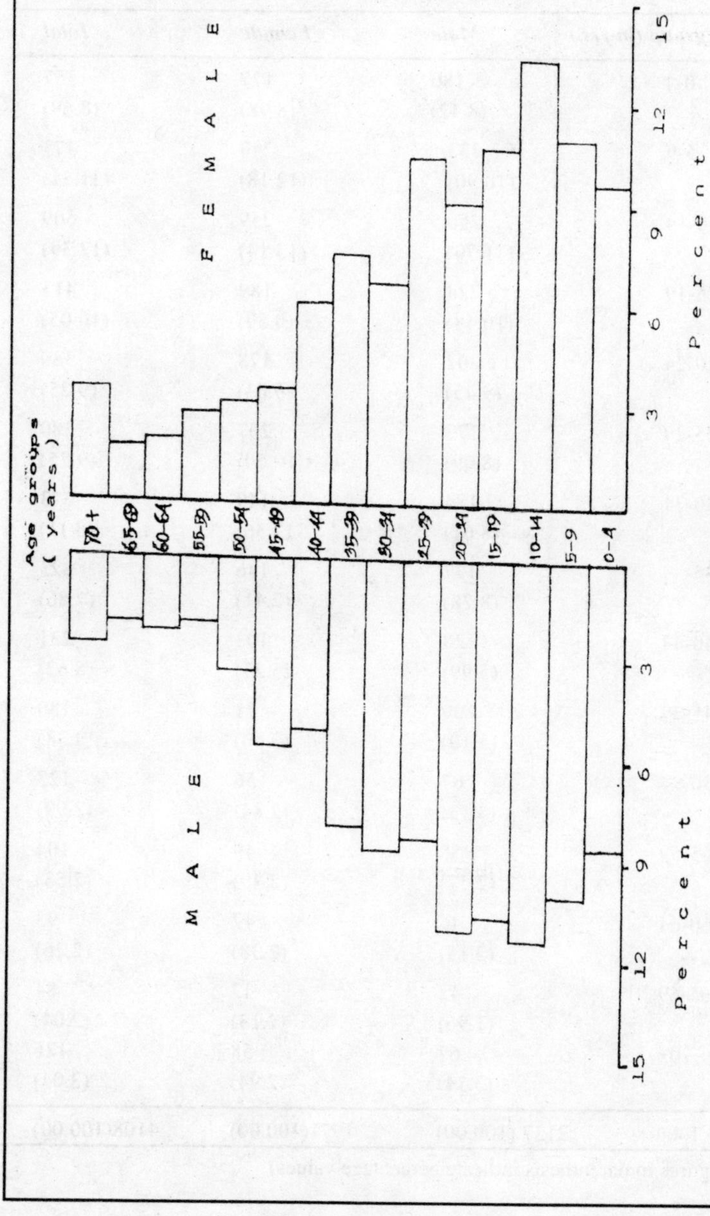

Fig.4.1 : Population Pyramid of the Namasudra

Table 4.1

Age-sex structure of the Namasudra population

Age group (in yrs.)	*Male*	*Female*	*Total*
0-4	180	177	357
	(8.42)	(8.98)	(8.69)
5-9	233	240	473
	(10.90)	(12.18)	(11.51)
10-14	250	259	509
	(11.70)	(13.14)	(12.39)
15-19	224	189	413
	(10.48)	(9.59)	(10.05)
20-24	202	178	380
	(9.45)	(9.03)	(9.25)
25-29	173	207	380
	(8.09)	(10.50)	(9.25)
30-34	184	149	333
	(8.61)	(7.56)	(8.11)
35-39	177	146	323
	(8.28)	(7.41)	(7.86)
40-44	128	103	231
	(5.99)	(5.23)	(5.62)
45-49	109	71	180
	(5.10)	(3.60)	(4.38)
50-54	67	56	123
	(3.13)	(2.84)	(2.99)
55-59	55	49	104
	(2.57)	(2.49)	(2.53)
60-64	46	47	93
	(2.15)	(2.38)	(2.26)
65-69	42	42	84
	(1.96)	(2.13)	(2.04)
70+	67	58	125
	(3.14)	(2.94)	(3.04)
Total	2137 (100.00)	1971(100.00)	4108(100.00)

(Figures in parenthesis indicate percentage values)

Table 4.1a

Age-sex structure of Namasudra population:Purana Bongaon

Age groups (in years)	*Village: Purana Bongaon*		
	Male	*Female*	*Total*
0-4	52 (10.87)	36 (8.45)	88 (9.73)
5-9	58 (12.13)	63 (14.79)	121 (13.39)
10-14	53 (11.09)	49 (11.50)	102 (11.28)
15-19	47 (9.83)	34 (7.98)	81 (8.96)
20-24	38 (7.95)	49 (11.50)	87 (9.62)
25-29	37 (7.74)	50 (11.74)	87 (9.62)
30-34	47 (9.83)	80 (9.39)	87 (9.62)
35-39	36 (7.53)	25 (5.87)	61 (6.73)
40-44	38 (7.95)	15 (3.52)	53 (5.86)
45-49	17 (3.56)	14 (3.29)	31 (3.43)
50-54	15 (3.14)	14 (3.29)	29 (3.21)
55-59	12 (2.15)	7 (1.64)	19 (2.10)
60-64	10 (2.09)	14 (3.29)	24 (2.65)
65-69	6 (1.26)	7 (1.64)	13 (1.44)
70+	12 (2.51)	9 (2.11)	21 (2.32)
Total	478 (99.63)	426 (100.00)	904 (99.96)

(Figures in parenthesis indicate percentage values)

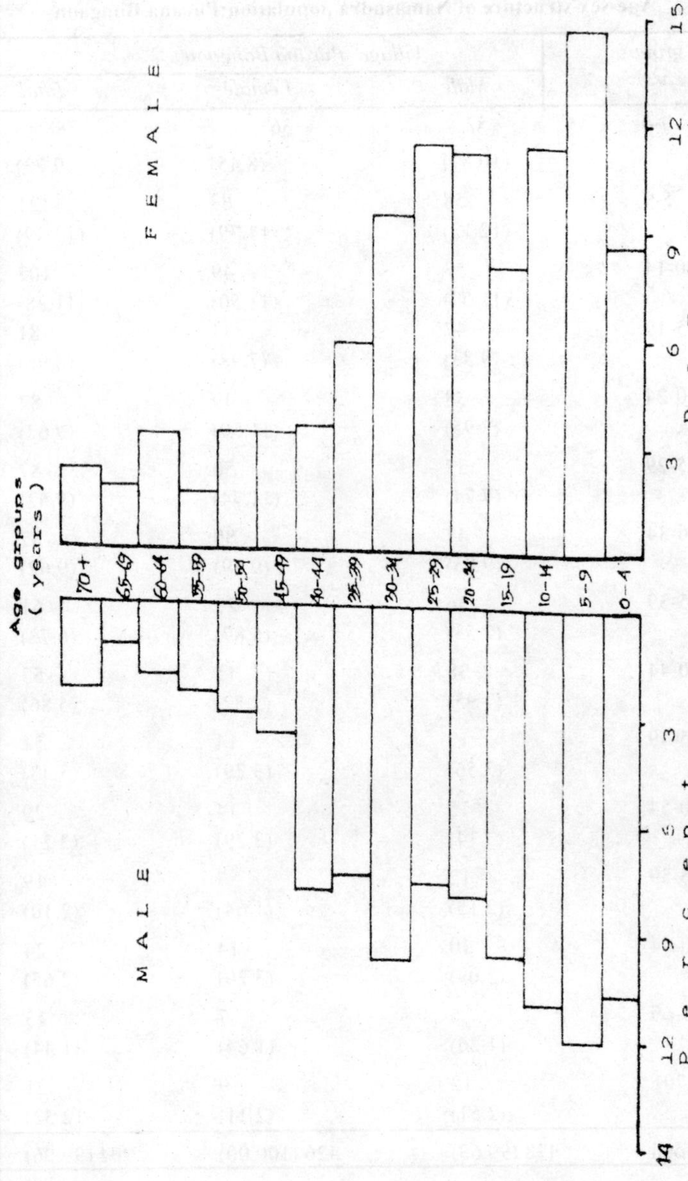

Fig.4.2 : Population Pyramid of the Namasudra : Purana Bangaon

Table 4.1b

Age-sex structure of Namasudra population: Paschim Ramchandrapur

Age groups (in years)	*Village: Paschim Ramchandrapur*		
	Male	*Female*	*Total*
0-4	89 (8.47)	95 (9.77)	184 (9.09)
5-9	106 (10.08)	107 (11.01)	213 (10.53)
10-14	118 (11.23)	130 (13.37)	248 (12.26)
15-19	113 (10.75)	104 (10.70)	217 (10.73)
20-24	117 (11.13)	88 (9.05)	205 (10.13)
25-29	88 (8.37)	100 (10.29)	188 (9.29)
30-34	91 (8.66)	63 (6.48)	154 (7.61)
35-39	85 (8.09)	72 (7.41)	157 (7.76)
40-44	54 (5.14)	58 (5.97)	112 (5.54)
45-49	59 (5.61)	33 (3.40)	92 (4.55)
50-54	36 (3.34)	29 (2.98)	65 (3.21)
55-59	22 (2.09)	26 (2.67)	48 (2.37)
60-64	23 (2.19)	18 (1.85)	41 (2.03)
65-69	22 (2.09)	16 (1.65)	38 (1.88)
70+	28 (2.66)	33 (3.40)	61 (3.01)
Total	**1051 (99.99)**	**972 (100.00)**	**2023 (99.99)**

(Figures in parenthesis indicate percentage values)

Of the total population 29.78 per cent males and 34.16 percent females fall in the age group 0-14 years, while in 15-49 years age group 57.75 per cent males and 53.29 percent females are recorded. The rest of the population falls in 50+ year's age group. However, in 10-14 years and 25-29 years age group considerably higher per cent of females are noticed than the males, while in 20-24 years age group a reverse trend is evident. Like village Purana Bongaon the population pyramid (Fig. 4.3) of the Namasudra of Paschim Ramchandrapur exhibits a progressive type population growth in the village.

Distribution of the Namasudra population according to age and sex is set out in Table 4.1c for village Kansona and in figure 4.4 the same has been presented in the form of population pyramid. Like other two villages in this village also a significant excess of males (51.48 %) relative to females (48.52 %) is noticed. It appears that there is a significant increase in number of individuals from 0-4 years to 5-9 years age group in both the sexes. However, from 5-9 years age group onwards a gradual decrease in the number of individuals is evident. This is true in both the sexes. Both the sexes share a more or less similar percent of individuals in all the age groups. Of the total population 30.76 per cent male and 34.2 per cent females fall in the age group 0-14 years, while in 15-49 years age group 54.28 per cent males and 52.01 percent females are recorded. The rest of the population falls in 50+ years age group. Like the population pyramid of other two villages, population pyramid of the Namasudra of Kansona village (Fig. 4.4) also suggests a trend of progressive type population growth. However, a constriction at the base of the population pyramid, suggests a recent fertility decline, or increased infant mortality.

Sex Ratio

For the purpose of present study, the sex ratio is defined as the number of males per hundred females. In Table 4.2 the sex-ratio values in the pre-reproductive (0-14 years), reproductive (15-49 years) and post-reproductive (50+ years) periods are presented for the Namasudra residing in three villages. It is interesting to note that in all these categories the males are always found to be excess

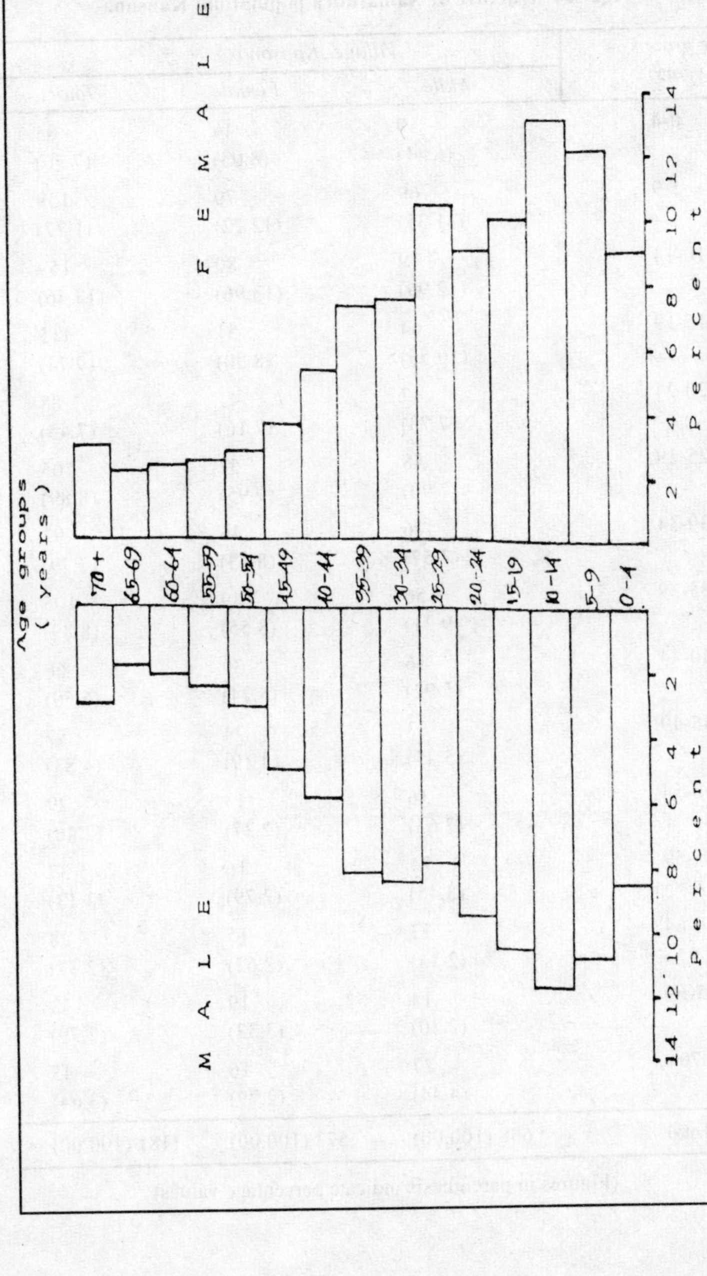

Fig.4.3 : Population Pyramid of the Namasudra :Paschim Ramchandrapur

Table 4.1c

Age-sex structure of Namasudra population: Kansona

Age groups (in years)	*Village: Kansona*		
	Male	*Female*	*Total*
0-4	39 (6.41)	46 (8.03)	85 (7.20)
5-9	69 (11.35)	70 (12.22)	139 (11.77)
10-14	79 (12.99)	80 (13.96)	159 (13.46)
15-19	64 (10.53)	51 (8.90)	115 (9.74)
20-24	47 (7.73)	41 (7.16)	88 (7.45)
25-29	48 (7.90)	57 (9.95)	105 (8.89)
30-34	46 (7.57)	46 (8.03)	92 (7.79)
35-39	56 (9.21)	49 (8.55)	105 (8.89)
40-44	36 (5.92)	30 (5.24)	66 (5.59)
45-49	33 (5.43)	24 (4.19)	57 (4.83)
50-54	16 (2.63)	13 (2.27)	29 (2.46)
55-59	21 (3.45)	16 (2.79)	37 (3.13)
60-64	13 (2.14)	15 (2.62)	28 (2.37)
65-69	14 (2.30)	19 (3.32)	33 (2.79)
70+	27 (4.44)	16 (2.79)	43 (3.64)
Total	608 (100.00)	573 (100.00)	1181 (100.00)

(Figures in parenthesis indicate percentage values)

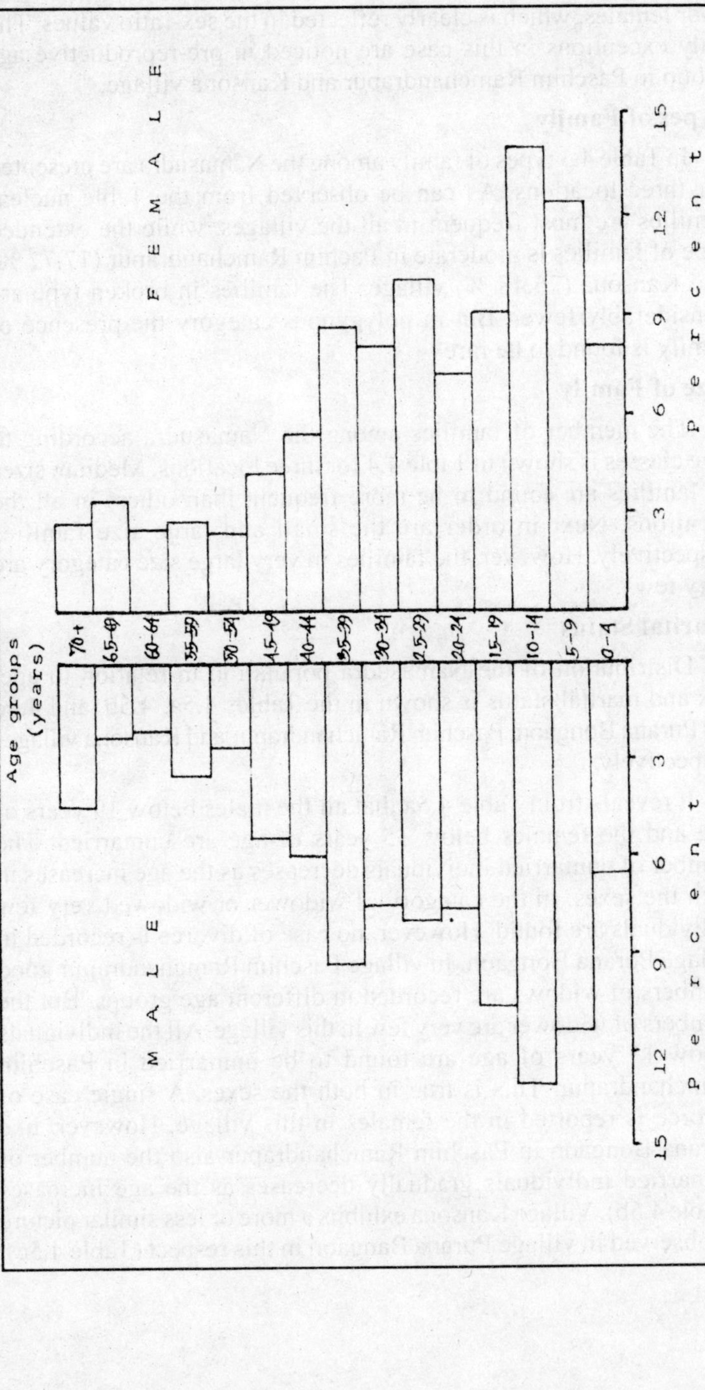

Fig.4.4 : Population Pyramid of the Namasudra : Kansona

over females, which is clearly reflected in the sex-ratio values. The only exceptions in this case are noticed in pre-reproductive age group in Paschim Ramchandrapur and Kansona village.

Types of Family

In Table 4.3 types of family among the Namasudra are presented for three locations. As can be observed from the Table nuclear families are most frequent in all the villages, while the extended type of families is moderate in Pachim Ramchandrapur (17.72 %) and Kansona (26.48 %) village. The families in broken type are considerably fewer. But in polygynous category the presence of family is found to be rare

Size of Family

The member of families among the Namasudra according to size classes is shown in Table 4.4 for three locations. Medium sizes of families are found to be more frequent than others in all the locations. Next in order are the small and large size families respectively. However, the families in very large size category are very few.

Marital Status

Distribution of the Namasudra population in relation to age, sex and marital status is shown in the Tables 4.5a, 4.5b, and 4.5c for Purana Bongaon, Paschim Ramchandrapur and Kansona villages respectively.

It reveals from Table 4.5a that all the males below 19 years of age and the females below 15 years of age are unmarried. The number of unmarried individuals decreases as the age increases in both the sexes. In the category of widower or widowed very few individuals are found. However, no case of divorce is recorded in village Purana Bongaon. In village Paschim Ramchandrapur good numbers of widows are recorded in different age groups. But the numbers of widower are very few in this village. All the individuals below 15 years of age are found to be unmarried in Paschim Ramchandrapur. This is true in both the sexes. A single case of divorce is reported in the females in this village. However, like Purana Bongaon in Paschim Ramchandrapur also the number of unmarried individuals gradually decreases as the age increases (Table 4.5b). Village Kansona exhibits a more or less similar picture as observed in village Purana Bangaon in this respect (Table 4.5c).

Table 4.2

Distribution of age, sex and sex-rations in pre-reproductive, reproductive and post-reproductive age groups among the Namasudra in three villages

Age group	*Purana Bongaon*			*Sex*	*Paschin Ramchandrapur*			*Sex*	*Kansona*			*Sex*
(in year)	*Male*	*Female*	*Total*	*Ratio*	*Male*	*Female*	*Total*	*Ratio*	*Male*	*Female*	*Total*	*Ratio*
Pre-Repro-ductive	163	148	311	110.13	313	332	645	94.28	187	196	383	95.41
(0–14)	(34.10)	(34.74)	(34.40)		(29.78)	(34.16)	(31.88)		(30.76)	(34.20)	(32.43)	
Reprod-uctive	260	227	487	114.54	607	518	1125	117.18	330	298	628	110.74
(15 – 49)	(54.39)	(53.29)	(53.87)		(57.75)	(53.29)	(55.61)		(54.28)	(52.01)	(53.18)	

Cont....

...Cont

Age group (in year)	Purana Bongaon			Sex Ratio	Paschin Ramchandrapur			Sex Ratio	Kansona			Sex Ratio
	Male	*Female*	*Total*		*Male*	*Female*	*Total*		*Male*	*Female*	*Total*	
Post-reproductive (50 +)	55 (11.51)	51 (11.97)	106 (11.73)	107.84	131 (12.46)	112 (12.55)	253 (12.51)	107.38	91 (14.96)	79 (13.79)	170 (14.39)	115.19
Total	478 (52.88)	426 (47.12)	904 (100.00)	112.21	1051 (51.95)	972 (48.05)	2023 (100.00)	108.13	608 (51.48)	573 (48.52)	1181 (100.00)	106.11

(Figures in parenthesis indicate percentage values)

Table 4.3

Types of family in three villages

Village	Nuclear family		Broken family		Extended family		Polygynous family		Total	
	No.	Percentage	No.	Percentage	No.	Percentage	No.	Percentage	No.	Percentage
Purana Bongaon	181	86.80	12	5.74	15	7.17	01	0.49	209	100.00
Paschim Ramchandrapur	298	75.44	26	6.58	70	17.72	01	0.26	295	100.00
Kansona	145	66.21	14	6.39	58	26.48	02	0.92	219	100.00
Grand Total	624	75.82	52	6.32	143	17.37	04	0.49	8.23	100.00

Table 4.4

Size of family in three villages

Location/ Village	*No. of Family*	*Small (< Members)*		*Medium (4-6 Members)*		*Large (7-9 Members)*		*Very Large (> 10 Members)*	
		No.	*Percentage*	*No.*	*Percentage*	*No.*	*Percentage*	*No.*	*Percentage*
Purana Boangaon	209	62	29.66	132	63.16	13	6.22	2	0.96
Paschim Ramchandrapur	395	80	20.25	235	59.49	63	15.94	17	4.32
Kansona	219	36	16.44	136	62.10	29	13.24	18	8.22
Total	823	178	21.61	503	61.29	105	1270	37	4.40

Table 4.5a

Distribution by age, sex and civil condition in Purana Bongaon village

Age groups	Males					Females				
(in Years)	Unmarried	Married	Widow	Divorced	Total	Unmarried	Married	Widow	Divorced	Total
10–14	163 (100.00)	–	–	–	163	148 (100.00)	–	–	–	148
15–19	47 (100.00)	–	–	–	47	24 (70.59)	10 (29.41)	–	–	34
20–24	28 (73.68)	10 (26.32)	–	–	38	6 (12.24)	42 (85.71)	1 (2.04)	–	49
25–29	13 (35.14)	24 (64.86)	–	–	37	4 (8.00)	46 (92.00)	–	–	50
30–34	7 (14.89)	40 (85.11)	–	–	47	–	38 (95.00)	2 (5.00)	–	40

Contd...

...Contd.

Age groups (in Years)	Males					Females				
	Unmarried	Married	Widow	Divorced	Total	Unmarried	Married	Widow	Divorced	Total
35–44	4 (5.41)	69 (93.24)	1 (1.35)	–	74	–	39 (97.50)	1 (2.50)	–	40
45–54	–	32 (100.00)	–	–	32	–	22 (78.57)	6 (21.43)	–	28
55–64	–	21 (95.45)	1 (4.55)	–	22	–	13 (61.90)	8 (38.10)	–	21
65+	–	16 (88.89)	2 (11.11)	–	18	–	2 (12.05)	14 (87.50)	–	16
Total	262 (54.81)	212 (44.35)	4 (0.84)	–	478 (100.00)	182 (42.72)	212 (49.77)	32 (7.51)	–	426 (100.00)

(Figures in parenthesis indicate percentage values)

Table 4.5b

Distribution by age, sex and civil condition in Paschim Ramchandrapur village

Age groups	Males					Females				
(in Years)	Unmarried	Married	Widow	Divorced	Total	Unmarried	Married	Widow	Divorced	Total
10–14	313 (100.00)	–	–	–	313	332 (100.00)	–	–	–	332
15–19	112 (99.11)	1 (0.88)	–	–	113	85 (81.73)	18 (17.31)	1 (0.96)	–	104
20–24	108 (92.30)	9 (7.69)	–	–	117	20 (22.73)	68 (77.27)	–	–	88
25–29	41 (46.59)	47 (53.41)	–	–	88	2 (2.00)	98 (98.00)	–	–	100

Contd...

...Contd.

Age groups	Males					Females				
(in Years)	Unmarried	Married	Widow	Divorced	Total	Unmarried	Married	Widow	Divorced	Total
30–34	11 (12.09)	79 (86.81)	1 (1.09)	–	91	2 (3.17)	58 (92.06)	3 (4.76)	–	63
35–44	4 (2.88)	135 (97.12)	–	–	139	1 (0.77)	116 (89.23)	12 (9.23)	1 (0.77)	130
45–54	1 (1.05)	94 (98.95)	–	–	95	–	51 (82.26)	11 (17.74)	–	62
55–64	–	41 (91.11)	4 (8.88)	–	45	–	34 (77.27)	10 (22.73)	–	44
65+	–	46 (92.00)	4 (8.00)	–	50	–	12 (24.49)	37 (75.51)	–	49
Total	590 (54.11)	452 (43.01)	9 (0.85)	–	1051 (100.00)	442 (45.47)	445 (46.81)	74 (7.61)	1 (0.10)	972 (100.00)

(Figures in parenthesis indicate percentage values)

Table 4.5c

Distribution by age, sex and civil condition in Kansona village

Age groups	Males					Females				
(in Years)	Unmarried	Married	Widow	Divorced	Total	Unmarried	Married	Widow	Divorced	Total
10-14	187 (100.00)	–	–	–	187	196 (100.00)	–	–	–	196
15–19	64 (100.00)	–	–	–	64	43 (84.31)	7 (13.73)	1 (1.96)	–	51
20–24	41 (87.23)	6 (12.77)	–	–	47	11 (26.83)	30 (73.17)	–	–	41
25–29	27 (56.25)	21 (43.75)	–	–	48	1 (1.75)	56 (98.25)	–	–	57
30–34	9 (19.57)	37 (80.43)	–	–	46	1 (2.17)	43 (93.48)	2 (4.35)	–	46

Contd...

...Contd.

Age groups	*Males*					*Females*				
(in Years)	*Unmarried*	*Married*	*Widow*	*Divorced*	*Total*	*Unmarried*	*Married*	*Widow*	*Divorced*	*Total*
35–44	–	92 (100.00)	–	–	92	–	72 (91.14)	7 (8.86)	–	79
45–54	–	49 (100.00)	–	–	49	–	32 (86.49)	5 (13.51)	–	37
55–64	–	34 (100.00)	–	–	34	–	22 (70.97)	9 (29.03)	–	31
65+	–	34 (82.93)	7 (17.07)	–	41	–	13 (37.14)	22 (62.86)	–	35
Total	328 (53.95)	273 (44.90)	7 (1.15)	–	608 (100.00)	252 (43.98)	275 (47.99)	46 (8.03)	–	573 (100.00)

(Figures in parenthesis indicate percentage values)

Table 4.6a

Educational status of the spouses in Purana Bongaon village

Age groups (in Years)	Husbands					Wives				
	Illiterate	Literates				Illiterate	Literates			
	Total	Primary (I –IV)	High School (V–X)	College (XI +)	Total	Total	Primary (I –IV)	High School (V–X)	College (XI +)	Total
15–19	–	–	–	–	–	1	4 (4.44)	4 (44.44)	1 (11.11)	9
20–24	3	2 (28.57)	5 (71.43)	–	7	11	7 (22.58)	22 (70.97)	2 (6.45)	31
25–29	4	5 (25.00)	15 (75.00)	–	20	17	9 (31.03)	20 (68.97)	–	29
30–34	12	7 (25.00)	14 (50.00)	7 (25.00)	28	12	6 (23.08)	20 (76.92)	–	26

Contd...

...Contd.

Age groups (in Years)	Husbands					Wives				
	Illiterate	Literates				Illiterate	Literates			
	Total	Primary (I–IV)	High School (V–X)	College (XI +)	Total	Total	Primary (I–IV)	High School (V–X)	College (XI +)	Total
35–44	14	18 (32.73)	28 (50.91)	9 (16.36)	55	15	10 (41.67)	14 (58.33)	–	24
45–54	5	9 (33.33)	15 (55.56)	3 (11.11)	27	10	3 (25.00)	9 (75.00)	–	12
55–64	5	4 (25.00)	12 (75.00)	–	16	6	3 (42.86)	4 (57.14)	–	7
65+	8	–	8 (100.00)	–	8	2	–	–	–	–
Total	51 (24.06)	45 (27.95)	97 (60.25)	19 (11.80)	161 (100.00)	74 (34.91)	42 (30.43)	93 (67.39)	3 (2.17)	138 (100.00)

(Figures in parenthesis indicate percentage values)

Table 4.6b

Educational status of the spouses in Paschim Ramchandrapur village

Age groups (in Years)	Husbands					Wives				
	Illiterate	Literates				Illiterate	Literates			
	Total	Primary (I –IV)	High School (V–X)	College (XI +)	Total	Total	Primary (I –IV)	High School (V–X)	College (XI +)	Total
15–19	1	–	–	–	–	2	4 (25.00)	12 (75.00)	–	16
20–24	1	2 (25.00)	5 (62.50)	1 (12.50)	8	9	5 (8.47)	50 (84.75)	4 (6.78)	59
25–29	10	12 (32.43)	23 (62.16)	2 (5.41)	37	22	18 (23.68)	55 (72.37)	3 (3.95)	76
30–34	15	12 (18.75)	43 (67.19)	9 (14.06)	64	19	10 (25.64)	26 (66.67)	3 (3.69)	39

Contd...

...Contd.

Age groups (in Years)	*Husbands*					*Wives*				
	Illiterate	*Literates*				*Illiterate*	*Literates*			
	Total	*Primary (I–IV)*	*High School (V–X)*	*College (XI +)*	*Total*	*Total*	*Primary (I–IV)*	*High School (V–X)*	*College (XI +)*	*Total*
35-44	26	20 (18.35)	76 (69.72)	13 (11.93)	109	36	28 (35.00)	48 (60.00)	4 (5.00)	80
45–54	23	18 (25.35)	41 (57.75)	12 (16.90)	71	23	12 (42.86)	16 (57.14)	–	28
55–64	15	5 (19.23)	20 (76.92)	1 (3.85)	26	18	10 (62.50)	6 (37.50)	–	16
65+	15	12 (38.71)	18 (58.06)	1 (3.23)	31	10	2 (100.00)	–	–	2
Total	106 (23.45)	81 (23.41)	226 (65.32)	39 (11.27)	346 (100.00)	139 (30.55)	89 (28.16)	213 (67.41)	14 (4.33)	316 (100.00)

(Figures in parenthesis indicate percentage values)

Table 4.6c

Educational status of the spouses in Kansona village

Age groups (in Years)	*Husbands*					*Wives*				
	Illiterate	*Literates*				*Illiterate*	*Literates*			
	Total	*Primary (I –IV)*	*High School (V–X)*	*College (XI +)*	*Total*	*Total*	*Primary (I –IV)*	*High School (V–X)*	*College (XI +)*	*Total*
15–19	–	–	–	–	–	–	1 (14.29)	6 (85.71)	–	7
20–24	2	2 (50.00)	2 (50.00)	–	4	9	–	21 (100.00)	–	21
25–29	3	3 (16.67)	15 (83.33)	–	18	12	6 (13.64)	34 (77.27)	4 (9.09)	44
30–34	4	6 (18.18)	20 (60.60)	7 (21.21)	33	17	8 (30.77)	18 (69.23)	–	26

Contd...

...Contd.

Age groups (in Years)	*Husbands*					*Wives*				
	Illiterate	*Literates*				*Illiterate*	*Literates*			
	Total	*Primary (I–IV)*	*High School (V–X)*	*College (XI +)*	*Total*	*Total*	*Primary (I–IV)*	*High School (V–X)*	*College (XI +)*	*Total*
35–44	18	10 (13.51)	52 (70.27)	12 (16.21)	74	36	11 (30.56)	24 (66.67)	1 (2.77)	36
45–54	16	6 (18.18)	25 (75.76)	2 (6.06)	33	14	18 (64.29)	9 (32.14)	1 (3.57)	28
55–64	6	12 (42.86)	14 (50.00)	2 (7.14)	28	19	1 (33.33)	2 (66.67)	–	3
65 +	17	3 (17.65)	13 (76.47)	1 (5.88)	17	2	1 (50.00)	1 (50.00)	–	2
Total	66 (24.17)	42 (20.29)	141 (68.12)	24 (11.59)	207 (100.00)	118 (42.91)	36 (22.93)	115 (73.25)	6 (3.82)	157 (100.00)

(Figures in parenthesis indicate percentage values)

Table 4.7

Occupation of the spouses in three villages

Type of Occupation	*Village*					
	Purana Bangaon		*Paschim Ramchandrapur*		*Kansona*	
	Male	*Female*	*Male*	*Female*	*Male*	*Female*
Agriculture	28	–	144	–	82	3
Agricultural Labour	1	–	–	–	–	–
Day Labour	52	–	96	–	70	3
Biri Binding	2	41	3	5	–	1
Hawker	18	–	–	–	11	–
Carpenter	14	–	–	–	2	–

Contd...

...Contd.

Type Of Occupation	*Village*					
	Purana Bangaon		*Paschim Ramchandrapur*		*Kansona*	
	Male	*Female*	*Male*	*Female*	*Male*	*Female*
Private Tutor	–	–	–	–	1	–
Driver	–	–	3	–	1	–
Teacher	1	–	4	3	–	2
Service	7	–	18	1	11	–
Chandsi Doctors/Com–pounder	2	–	11	–	21	–
Business	41	–	115	2	40	1
Tailor	3	–	4	–	1	–

...Contd.

Type of Occupation	*Village*					
	Purana Bangaon		*Paschim Ramchandrapur*		*Kansona*	
	Male	*Female*	*Male*	*Female*	*Male*	*Female*
Van/Rickshaw Puller	32	–	18	–	5	–
Snake Charmer	1	–	–	–	–	–
Weaving	–	–	–	–	1	1
Retired Person	–	–	10	–	2	–
Total	202	41	426	11	248	11
Percentage	100.00	20.50			100.00	

Educational Status

Educational status of the Namasudra spouses is shown in Tables 4.6a, 4.6b, and 4.6c respectively for the three villages. It reveals from the tables that the wives outnumber the husbands in illiteracy. While the percent of illiterate husbands ranges between 23.45 and 24.17, the percent of illiterate wives ranges between 3.55 and 42.91 in three villages. Village Kansona exhibits highest percent of illiterate husbands (24.17) and wives (42.91). Side by side, village Paschim Ramchandrapur exhibits lowest percent of illiterate husbands (23.45) and wives (30.55). Difference in number of illiterate husbands is found to be very low in three villages. In respect of primary, high school and college level education a more or less similar trend is noticed in three villages. This is true for both the sexes. However, the percent of college level educated wives are found to be considerably lower than that of the husbands, which again is recorded to be lowest in the village Kansona (Table 4.6c)

Occupational Status

Occupational status of the spouses is shown for three villages (Table 4.7). It reveals that in Purana Bongaon most of the husbands are engaged in daily labour, business and rickshaw pulling job, while one fifth of the wives are found to be engaged in bidi binding job in this. In Paschim Ramchandrapur village most of the husbands are engaged in day labour and business. But in Kansona a good number of husbands are engaged in own agriculture along with day labour and business. However, few numbers of wives are found to be engaged in different kinds of job in these two villages.

5

REPRODUCTIVE PERFORMANCE

Reproductive patterns vary between two cultural groups, between communities of various socioeconomic status even communities residing in different geographical settings. Rele (1982) says that the survival and growth of any family or a closed social group depends intrinsically upon the level of fertility in relation to mortality. We shall deal various aspects of reproductive performance among the Namasudra residing in Purana Bongaon, Paschim Ramchandrapur and Kansona village in this chapter.

Altogether four twin births have been found among them. Out of thses two cases of twins are recorded in Purana Bongaon village. Side by side, in Kansona village also two cases are reported. But in Paschim Ramchandrapur there is no such case. Altogether there are three married women, who are found to be sterile. Out of these three married women one belong to Purana Bongaon village and the rest other two belong to Kansona village. In Table 5.1 number of mothers are shown according to villages. Altogether, 876 mothers are taken into consideration for the purpose of present study. Out of which 202 belong to Purana Bongaon village and 426 belong to Paschim Ramchandrapur village, while the rest i.e. 248 mothers belong to village Kansona.

Table 5.1

Number of mothers according to villages

Village	*Total number of mothers*
Purana Bongaon	202
Paschim Ramchandrapur	426
Kansona	248
Total	876

Age specific occurrence of menarche has been presented for the Namasudra in Table 5.2 and the same is presented for three villages in Table 5.2a. Maximum occurrence of menarche is recorded in 13 years of age, which is true for the Namasudra residing the three different villages. However, in 12 and 14 years of age a good percent of them are recorded.

Table 5.2

Age specific occurrence of menarche among the Namasudra women

Age at menarche (in years)	*No.*	*Percentage*
11	56	6.39
12	154	17.58
13	349	39.89
14	117	13.36
15	83	9.47
16	56	6.39
17	23	2.63
18	24	2.74
19	14	1.60
Total	876	99.99

Table 5.2a

Age specific occurrence of menarche according to villages

Age at Menarche (in Years)	*Purana Bongaon*		*Paschim Ramchandrapur*		*Kansona*	
	No.	*%*	*No.*	*%*	*No.*	*%*
11	11	5.44	27	6.34	11	4.43
12	35	17.33	69	16.20	44	17.74
13	80	39.60	165	38.73	95	38.31
14	27	13.37	61	14.32	38	15.32
15	19	9.41	42	9.86	26	10.48
16	13	6.44	32	7.51	16	6.45
17	6	2.97	9	2.11	6	2.42
18	8	3.96	9	2.11	7	2.82
19	3	1.48	12	2.82	5	2.02
Total	**202**	**100.00**	**426**	**100.00**	**248**	**99.99**

Table 5.3

Age-specific occurrence of menopause among the Namasudra women

Age at menopause (in years)	*No.*	*%*
41	5	2.07
42	6	2.49
43	13	5.39
44	16	6.64
45	31	12.86
46	51	21.16
47	48	19.92
48	27	11.20
49	26	10.79
50	18	7.47
Total	**241**	**99.99**

Age specific occurrence of menopause has been presented for the Namasudra in Table 5.3, while the same has been presented village-wise in Table 5.3a. Altogether 241 women were found among the Namasudra who attained their menstruation. In Purana Bongaon, Paschim Ramchandrapur and Kansona their numbers are 45, 120 and 76 respectively. It reveals that most of them have attained their menopause at the age of 46 years. Side by side, a good number of them are also found in 45 and 47 years in this respect. This is true among the Namasudra residing in three villages.

Table 5.3a

Age-specific occurrence of menopause according to villages

Age at menopause	*Purana Bongaon*		*Paschim Ramchandrapur*		*Kansona*	
(in years)	*No.*	*%*	*No.*	*%*	*No.*	*%*
41	–	–	2	1.67	–	–
42	1	2.22	–	–	2	2.63
43	–	–	–	–	–	–
44	4	8.89	10	8.33	7	9.21
45	8	17.78	26	21.67	16	21.05
46	10	22.22	28	23.33	18	23.68
47	8	17.78	21	17.5	12	15.79
48	6	13.33	15	12.50	8	10.53
49	5	11.11	12	10.00	7	9.21
50	3	6.67	6	5.00	6	7.89
Total	45	100.00	120	100.00	76	99.99

Reproductive performance of the post-menopausal women is furnished for the Namasudra in Table 5.4, while the same has been according to villages in Table 5.4a.

It reveals that there is an u-turn in average live births with the increase in age at menarche among the studied population. Average live births are enumerated to be highest among the women who attained their menarche in 13-14 years age group and the lowest is recorded in 15 years and above age group. While, in 11-12 years age group an intermediate value is recorded in this respect (Table 5.4). A more or less similar trend is noticed in case of three villages (Table 5.4a). However, average numbers of deaths are found to be increasing with the increase in age at menarche among the study population (Table 5.4), which is true for the Namasudra residing in Kansona village. But in Purana Bongaon and Paschim Ramchandrapur village a dissimilar trend is noticed. In Purana Bongaon village lowest average of deaths is recorded in 13-14 years age group while in Paschim Ramchandrapur the same is recorded in 15 years and above age group (Table 5.4a).

Table 5.4

Reproductive performance of post-menopausal Namasudra women

Age at menarche (in years)	*No. of mothers*	*Average no. of pregnancies*	*Average no. of deaths*	*Average live births*
11-12	57	6.32	0.13	6.01
13-14	111	6.34	0.14	6.12
15 & above	73	5.81	0.25	5.43
Total	241	6.21	0.18	5.86

Average numbers of live births of all the mothers are presented in Table 5.5 according to villages. It is interesting to note that average number of live births per mother increases in these villages as the geographical distance increases from the Block head quarter. Average number is recorded to be lowest in Purana Bongaon village (3.0841 ± 0.1323) and highest in Kansona village (3.7137 ± 0.1500), whereas in Paschim Ramchandrapur village (3.5446 ± 0.1060) an intermediate value is recorded.

Table 5.4a

Reproductive performance of post-menopausal women according to villages

Age at Menarche (in years)	*Purana Bongaon*			*Paschim Ramchandrapur*			*Kansona*		
	No. of mothers	*Average no. of deaths*	*Average live births*	*No. of mothers*	*Average no. of deaths*	*Average live births*	*No. of mothers*	*Average no. of deaths*	*Average live births*
11-12	9	0.14	5.89	27	0.12	6.01	19	0.14	6.02
13-14	23	0.12	6.17	54	0.32	6.34	34	0.28	6.72
15 & above	13	0.21	5.34	39	0.14	5.81	23	0.25	5.78
Total	45	0.16	5.87	120	0.19	6.05	76	0.23	6.16

Table 5.5

Average live births according to villages

Village births	*No. of mothers*	*Total no. of live birih*	*Average live births per mother ± S.E*
Purana Bongaon	202	623	3.0841 ± 0.1323
Paschim Ramchandrapur	426	1510	3.5446 ± 0.1060
Kansona	248	921	3.7137 ± 0.1500
Total	876	3054	3.4863 ± 0.1231

In Tables 5.6a, 5.6b and 5.6c, the number of live births and surviving children of the mothers by age groups, have been given for the Namasudra residing in Purana Bongaon, Paschim Ramchandrapur and Kansona village respectively. It is seen that the mean of live births and surviving children in all the villages increases with the advancement of mother's age. In Purana Bongaon village, the average number of live births increases from 1.1667 ± 0.1521 for the mothers in 15-19 years age group to 5.3158 ± 0.3268 for the mothers aged 45 years above. Side by side, the average number of surviving children increases from 1.1667 ± 0.1521 for the mothers in 15-19 years age group to 4.2368 ± 0.2917 for the mothers aged 45 years and above in this village (Table 5.4a). The average number of live births in Paschim Ramchandrapur village is found to be comparatively lower among the mothers in 15-19 years age group (1.3333 ± 0.2722) than village Purana Bangaon (1.6667 ± 0.1521). But in 45 years and above age group the mean number of live births is recorded to be considerably higher in Paschim Ramchandrapur (6.1584 ± 0.2071) than village Purana Bangaon (5.3158 ± 0.3268). In case of surviving children, however, a more or less similar trend is evident (Table 5.4b). Whereas, in Kansona village mean number of live births increases from 1.0000 for the mothers in 15-19 years age group to 6.1323 ± 0.3174 for the mothers in 45 years and above age group. Side by side, the average number of surviving children increases from 1.0000 for the mothers in 15-19 years age group to 4.8529 ± 0.2480 for the

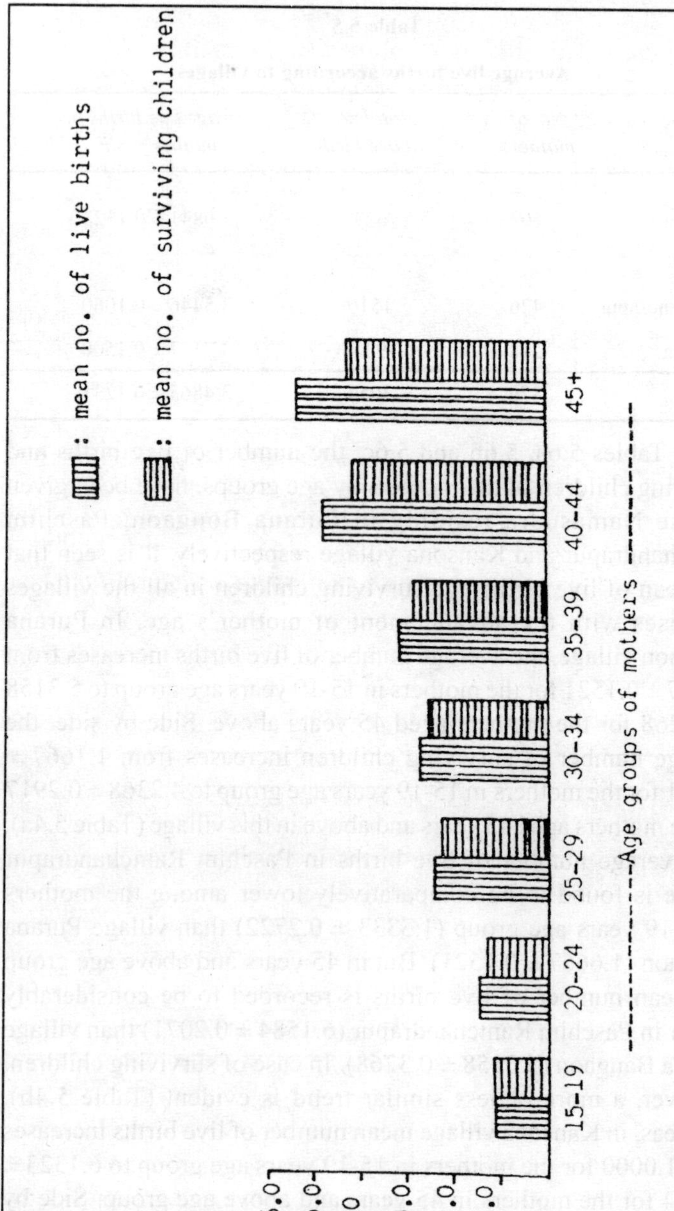

Fig. 5.1: Average live births and surviving children by age groups of mothers : Purana Bongaon

Table 5.6a

Live births and surviving children according to age groups of the mothers in Purana Bongaon village

Age Groups (in years)	*No. of mothers*	*Total no. of live births*	*No. of surviving children*	*Average no. of live births ± S.E*	*Average no. of live surviving children ± S.E*
15-19	6	7	7	1.1667 ± 0.1521	1.1667 ± 0.1521
20-24	38	54	49	1.4210 ± 0.1213	1.2895 ± 0.1229
25-29	41	100	92	2.4390 ± 0.1620	2.2439 ± 0.1572
30-34	36	99	92	2.7500 ± 0.1816	2.5555 ± 0.1493
35-39	29	92	81	3.1724 ± 0.2442	2.7931 ± 0.1645
40-44	14	68	58	4.8571 ± 0.3171	4.1429 ± 0.3171
45+	38	203	161	5.3158 ± 0.3268	4.2368 ± 0.2917
Total	202	623	540	3.0841 ± 0.2331	2.6733 ± 0.1378

Table 5.6b

Live births and surviving children according to age groups of the mothers in Paschim Ramchandrapur village

Age Groups (in years)	*No. of mothers*	*Total no. of live births*	*No. of surviving children*	*Average no. of live births ± S.E*	*Average no. of live surviving children ± S.E*
15-19	3	4	4	1.3333±0.2722	1.3333±0.2722
20-24	57	93	85	2.0000±0.3868	1.4912±0.1085
25-29	94	206	189	2.1915±0.1234	2.0106±0.1111
30-34	55	158	148	2.8727±0.1522	2.6909±0.1452
35-39	65	208	179	3.2000±0.1430	2.7538±0.1324
40-44	51	219	192	4.5686±0.3444	3.7647±0.2011
45+	101	622	519	6.1584±0.2071	5.1386±0.1771
Total	426	1510	1316	3.5446±0.1488	3.0892±0.1457

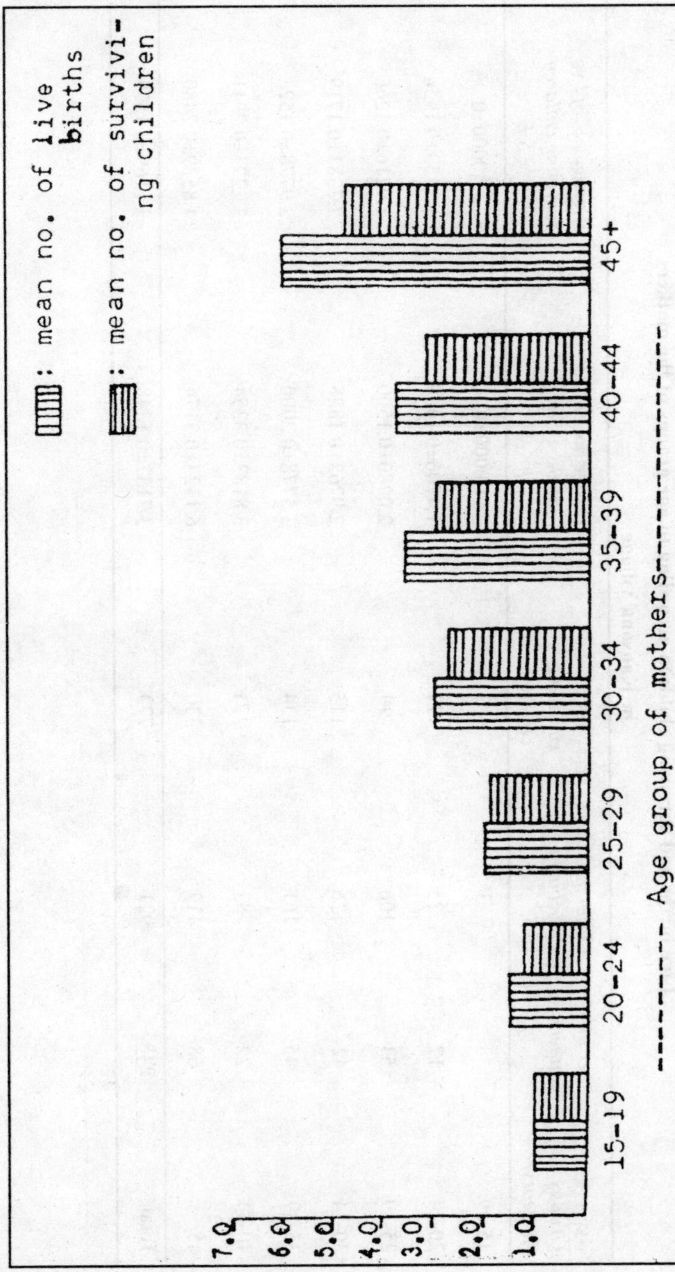

Fig. 5.2: Average live births and surviving chldren by age groups of mothers : Paschim Ramchandrapur

Table 5.6c

Live births and surviving children according to age groups of the mothers in Kansona village

Age Groups (in years)	*No. of mothers*	*Total no. of live births*	*No. of surviving children*	*Average no. of live births ± S.E*	*Average no. of live surviving children ± S.E*
15-19	3	3	3	1.0000±0	1.0000±0
20-24	17	25	21	1.4706±0.1469	1.2353±0.1956
25-29	51	106	99	2.0980±0.1500	1.9216±0.1266
30-34	42	126	115	2.9762±0.1828	2.7381±0.1719
35-39	45	161	134	3.5778±0.2000	2.9778±0.1523
40-44	22	83	71	3.8182±0.3254	3.2273±0.2941
45+	68	417	330	6.1323±0.3174	4.8529±0.2480
Total	248	921	773	3.7137±0.1348	3.1169±0.1579

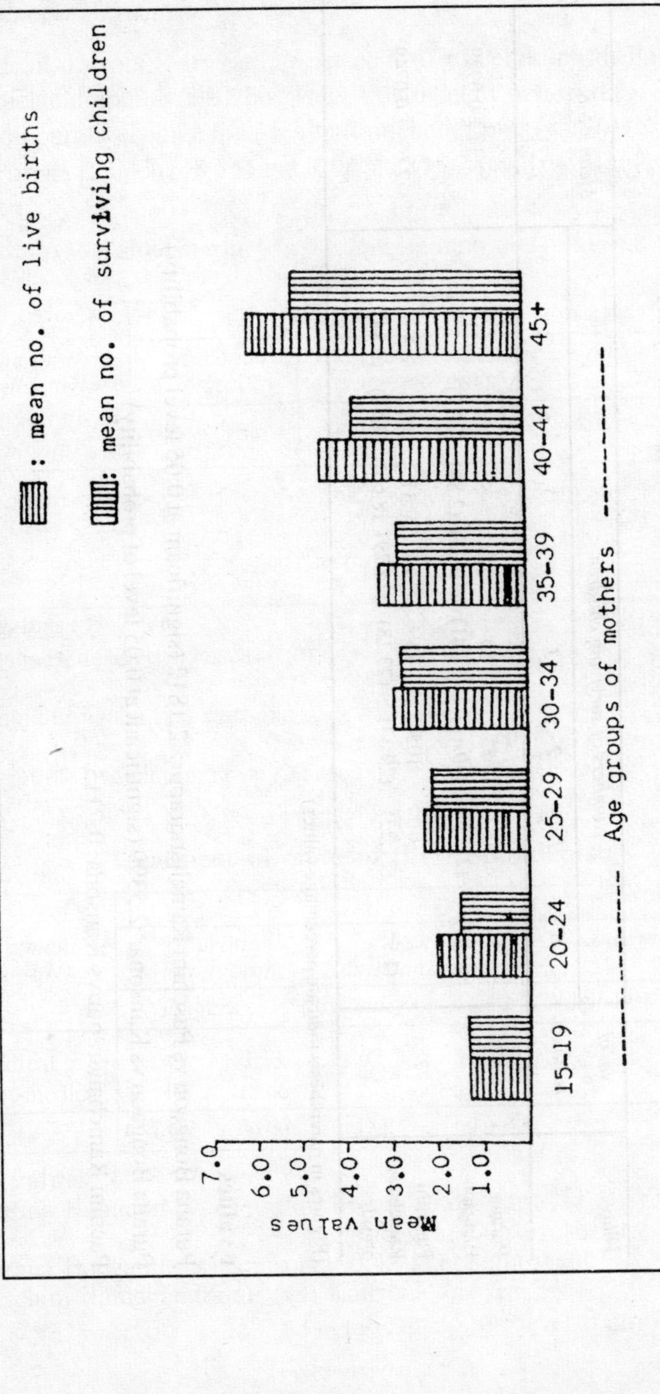

Fig. 5.3: Average live births and surviving chldren by age groups of mothers : Kansona

Table 5.7

Surviving sibship size among the married women aged 15-49 years

Village	*No. of mothers*	*Numbers of surviving children*									*Mean ± S.E.*
		0	*1*	*2*	*3*	*4*	*5*	*6*	*7*	*8*	
Purana Bangaon	176	5 (2.84)	41 (23.29)	53 (30.11)	50 (28.41)	18 (10.23)	5 (2.84)	4 (2.27)	–	–	2.37 ± 0.0929
Paschim Ramchan-drapur	358	7 (1.95)	76 (21.23)	105 (29.33)	83 (23.18)	44 (12.29)	31 (8.66)	9 (2.51)	3 (0.84)	–	2.63 ± 0.0749

(Figures in parenthesis indicate percentage values)

t values :

Purana Bongaon vs Paschim Ramchandrapur: 2.1812 (significant at 0.05 level probability)

Purana Bongaon vs Kansona: 2.5399 (significant at 0.05 level of probability)

Pachim Ramchandrapur vs Kansona: 0.7115

mothers in 45 years and above age group (Table 5.4c). This reflects a more or less similar trend with village Paschim Ramchandrapur. Mean number of live births and surviving children according to mothers age are presented in figures 5.1, 5.2 and 5.3 graphically for the villages Purana Bongaon, Paschim Ramchandrapur and Kansona respectively.

Numbers of married women of active reproductive period (i.e. 15-49 years) and surviving sibship size are shown in Table 5.7 for three villages. Mean number of surviving children increases from Purana Bongaon (2.37 ± 0.0929) to Kansona (2.72 ± 0.1020) through Paschim Ramchandrapur village (2.63 ± 0.0749), indicative of fertility increment with the increment in geographic distance from urban centre. The difference between Purana Bongaon and Paschim Ramchandrapur (t = 2.1812), and Purana Bongaon and Kansona (t = 2.5399) is statistically significant. But the difference between Paschim Ramchandrapur and Kansona (t = 0.7115) is not statisticaily significant in this respect. It is also found that highest percent of mothers have two number of surviving children. This is true for the mothers residing in all the three villages.

In Table 5.8 average live births of the Namasudra women is presented according to the age at marriage. It reveals that average of live births decreases with the increase in age at marriage, which is true for all the villages. However, the average live birth is found to be comparatively lower in Purana Bongaon village than other two villages. Side by side, these values are comparatively lower in Paschim Ramchandrapur than that of Kansona village.

Infant mortality for the Namasudra residing in three villages are presented in Table 5.9. It is interesting to note that like average live births in case of infant mortality also the percentage values increases in the villages as their geographical distance from the nearest urban centre increases. Infant mortality is found to be 5.07 percent among the Namasudra. When the three villages are taken into consideration it is found to be lowest in Purana Bongaon (3.85 percent) and highest in Kansona villages (6.30 percent), whereas in Paschim Ramchandrapur village an intermediate value (4.83 percent) is recorded. It is, however,

Table 5.8

Age at marriage and average live births among the Namasudra women

Age of marriage (in years)	*Purana Bongaon*		*Paschim Ramchandrapur*		*Kansona*		*Total*	
	No. of mothers	*Average live births*	*No. of mothers*	*Average live births*	*No. of mothers*	*Average live birth*	*No. of mothers*	*Average live birth*
-19	37	3.79	68	3.95	49	4.10	176	3.89
20-24	158	3.11	347	3.31	196	3.95	668	3.33
25 & above	7	2.41	11	2.37	3	2.78	32	2.31
Total	202	3.10	426	3.21	248	3.61	876	3.17

interesting to note that in Kansona village the percent of infant mortality is recorded to be much higher than Purana Bongaon and Paschim Ramchandrapur village.

In Table 5.10 percent of toddler (1-4 years) and under-5 mortality are presented. Percent of toddler and under-5 mortality are 1.80 and 6.88 respectively among the Namasudra. Like infant mortality in case of toddler and under-5 mortality a similar trend is noticed. However, in Kansona village both the toddler and under-5 mortality are found to be much higher than other two villages.

Pregnancy wastage among the Namasudra is shown in Table 5.11 for three villages. This percentage value is recorded to be highest in Paschim Ramchandrapur (2.17) and lowest in Purana Bongaon village (1.58). In village Kansona, however, slightly lower percent (2.54) of pregnancy wastage is recorded than that of village Paschim Ramchandrapur. When the mean number of conception is taken into consideration lowest average is recorded in village Purana Bongaon (3.13) and highest is in village Kansona (3.81), whereas village Paschim Ramchandrapur stands in between (3.64) in this respect.

Like pregnancy wastage in case of perinatal mortality also the highest percent is recorded in Paschim Ramchandrapur village (5.48) and lowest is in Purana Bongaon village (2.37). In village Kansona slightly lower percent of perinatal mortality (5.29) is recorded than that of village PaschimRamchandrapur. However, this percentage value is found to be less than half in Purana Bongaon village than other two villages. When these percentage values are combined together the percent of perinatal mortality among the Namasudra is found to be 4.79 (Table 5.12).

When the binomial test of equality of proportion is performed for infant, toddler and under-5 mortality in three villages it is found that there is significant difference between village Purana Bongaon and Kansona in case of these three mortalities. Side by side between Paschim Ramchandrapur and Kansona significant difference is noticed in case of toddler and under-5 mortality. But between Purana Bongaon and Paschim Ramchandrapur there is no significant difference in case of all three mortalities (Table 5.13).

Table 5.9

Infant mortality according to villages

Village	*No. of mothers*	*Total no. of live births*	*Neonatal deaths*	*Post neonatal deaths*	*Total infant deaths*	*Infant mortality (in %)*
Purana Bongaon	202	623	5 (0.80)	19 (3.05)	24	3.85
Paschim Ramchandra-pur	426	1510	43 (2.85)	30 (1.99)	73	4.83
Kansona	248	921	26 (2.82)	32 (3.47)	58	6.30
Total	876	3054	74 (2.42)	81 (2.65)	155	5.07

(Figures in parenthesis indicate percentage values)

Table 5.10

Child mortality according to villages

Village	*No. of mothers*	*Total no. of live births*	*Toddler mortality (1-4 years)*	*Toddler mortality (in %)*	*Under-5 mortality*	*Under-5 mortality (in %)*
Purana Bongaon	202	623	7	1.12	31	4.97
Paschim Ramchan-drapur	426	1510	19	1.26	92	6.09
Kansona	248	921	29	3.15	87	9.45
Total	876	3054	55	1.80	210	6.88

Table 5.11

Pregnancy wastage according to villages

Village	*No. of mothers*	*No. of conceptions*	*Mean conception*	*No. of abortion*	*No. of still birth*	*Total pregnancy wastage*	*Pregnancy wastage (in %)*
Purana Bongaon	202	633	3.13	3 (0.47)	7 (1.11)	10	1.58
Paschim Ramchandra-pur	426	1552	3.64	29 (1.87)	13 (0.84)	42	2.71
Kansona	248	945	3.81	11 (1.16)	13 (1.38)	24	2.54
Total	876	3130	3.57	43 (1.37)	33 (1.05)	76	2.43

(Figures in parenthesis indicate percentage values)

ASSOCIATION OF SOCIO-CULTURAL FACTORS WITH FERTILITY AND INFANT MORTALITY

In this section some socio-cultural factors such as mother's education, socio-economic status, type of family, size of family and age at marriage are taken into consideration to examine their association with fertily and infant mortality among the study population.

Mother's education, fertility and infant mortality

It reveals from Table 5.14 that average live births and percent of infant mortality decreases as the level of education increase in the study population. This is true for all the three villages. A low level of fertility and infant mortality is however, recorded in Purana Bongaon village than other two villages.

Economic status, and fertility and infant mortality

It reveals from Table 5.15 that the level of fertility and infant mortality increases as the level of income decreases among the study population. This is true for the Namasudra residing in three villages. The only exception in this respect is noticed in case of the mothers belong to the middle-income status families in Paschmi Ramchandrapur village. Thus there exists an inverse relationship between income, and fertility and infant mortality.

Type of family, and fertility and infant mortality

It reveals from Table 5.16 that in resect of type of family and fertily and infant mortality no such definite trend is noticed among the Namasudra. This is true for the study population residing in three villages.

Size of family, and fertility and infant mortality

It is seen from Table 5.17 that fertility and infant mortality increases from nuclear to large size of families through medium size families. This is true for the Namasudra residing in three villages. The exceptions of this trend are noticed in case of average live births in Purana Bongaon and Paschim Ramchandrapur village.

Age at marriage and infant mortality

In Table 5.18 age at marriage of the Namasudra is examined in terms of infant mortality. This is to be noted that age at marriage and fertility is examined earlier among the study population, which is presented in Table 5.8. It reveals from Table 5.18 that highest percent of infant deaths occurred among the mothers who married at an early age (i.e. below 20 years). Side by side, the same is evident among the mothers who married at an late age (i.e. 25

Table 5.12

Perinatal mortality according to villages

Village	*No. of mothers*	*No. of conceptions*	*Total pregnancy wastage*	*Total neo-natal deaths*	*Perinatal deaths*	*Perinatal mortality (in %)*
Purana Bongaon Paschim	202	633	10 (1.58)	5 (0.79)	15	2.37
Ramchandrapur	426	1552	42 (2.71)	43 (2.77)	85	5.48
Kansona	248	945	24 (2.54)	26 (2.75)	50	5.29
Total	876	3130	76 (2.43)	74 (2.36)	150	4.79

(Figures in parenthesis indicate percentage values)

Table 5.13
Binomial test of equality of proportion on infant, toddler and under – 5 mortality

Village	*Infant mortality*			*Toddler mortality*			*Under – 5 mortality*		
	Ti	***T_2***	*Inference*	***Ti***	***T_2***	*Inference*	***Ti***	***T_2***	*Inference*
Purana Bongaon Vs Paschim Ramchandrapur	0.0098	0.0100	NS*	0.0014	0.0052	NS*	0.0112	0.0111	NS*
Purana Bongaon Vs Kansona	0.0245	0.0116	S**	0.0203	0.0078	S**	0.0447	0.0138	S**
Paschim Ramchandrapur Vs Kansona	0.0147	0.0096	NS*	0.0189	0.0059	S**	0.0336	0.0111	S**

* N.S. = Not significant
**S = Significant

Table 5.14

Impact of mother's education on fertility and infant mortality

Mother's education	*Village*									*Total*		
	Purana Bongaon			*Paschim Ramchadrapur*			*Kansona*					
	No. of Mothers	*Average live births*	*Infant mortality (in %)*	*No. of mothers*	*Average live births*	*Infant mortality (in %)*	*No. of mothers*	*Average live births*	*Infant mortality (in %)*	*No. of mothers*	*Average live births*	*Infant mortality (in %)*
Illiterate	73	4.19	4.48	139	4.78	5.78	118	5.43	6.01	330	4.78	6.23
Primary level	93	3.29	3.37	213	3.56	4.98	115	4.58	4.45	421	4.34	5.45
High School & above	36	2.98	3.01	74	3.01	3.72	15	3.78	3.82	125	3.23	3.98

Table 5.15:
Impact of economic status on fertility and infant mortality

Economic status	Village									Total		
	Purana Bongaon			Paschim Ramchandrapur			Kansona					
	No. of mothers	Average live births	Infant mortality (in%)	No. of mothers	Average live births	Infant mortality (in %)	No. of mothers	Average live births	Infant mortlity (in%)	No.of mothers	Average live births	Infant mortality (in%)
High	38	3.33	3.78	76	3.35	4.08	21	3.69	4.59	135	3.23	4.31
Medium	95	3.81	4.01	216	3.23	4.78	118	4.83	5.78	429	4.37	5.25
Low	69	4.23	4.25	134	4.79	5.41	109	5.01	6.72	312	5.38	6.01

Table 5.16

Impact of type of family on fertility and infant mortality

Type of Family	Village									Total		
	Purana Bongaon			Paschim Ramchadrapur			Kansona					
	No. of Mothers	Average live births	Infant mortality (in %)	No. of mothers	Average live births	Infant mortality (in %)	No. of mothers	Average live births	Infant mortality (in %)	No. of mothers	Average live births	Infant mortality (in %)
Nuclear	175	4.01	4.01	298	4.78	4.23	145	4.95	4.78	618	5.38	4.38
Broken	12	3.78	3.25	42	3.25	5.01	35	5.73	5.32	89	5.47	5.78
Joint	15	3.49	3.71	86	4.32	5.37	68	5.02	5.29	169	5.58	5.49

Table 5.17

Impact of size of family on fertility and infant mortality

Size of family	*Village*									*Total*		
	Purana Bongaon			*Paschim Ramchadrapur*			*Kansona*					
	No. of Mothers	*Average live births*	*Infant mortality (in %)*	*No. of mothers*	*Average live births*	*Infant mortality (in %)*	*No. of mothers*	*Average live births*	*Infant mortality (in %)*	*No. of mothers*	*Average live births*	*Infant mortality (in %)*
Small	62	4.03	4.74	80	4.63	4.83	36	4.85	4.37	178	5.37	5.78
Medium	92	3.70	4.82	225	3.83	5.29	160	4.98	5.28	477	4.78	5.28
Large	48	3.35	4.27	121	3.71	5.28	52	5.78	5.82	221	5.25	5.31

Table 5.18

Effect of age at marriage on infant mortality

Age at marriage (in years)	Village						Total	
	Purana Bongaon		Paschim Ramchadrapur		Kansona			
	No. of Mothers	Infant mortality (in %)	No. of mothers	Infant mortality (in %)	No. of mothers	Infant mortality (in %)	No. of mothers	Infant mortality (in %)
– 19	37	4.03	68	5.03	49	6.12	176	5.85
20-24	158	3.21	347	4.09	196	4.79	668	4.93
25 & above	7	3.32	11	4.49	3	5.03	32	5.48

6

HEALTH CARE PRACTICES

Concept of Health, Perception and Treatment of Diseases:

In order to collect necessary information on concept of health among the study population 90 elderly individuals from the three villages were interviewed. In this connection thirty individuals were randomly selected from each village.

It appears that 60 per cent of the respondents are able to define the term "health". According to majority of them, a healthy person can be defined, as "one who is able to perform his/her daily or routine work properly and he/she must not be suffering from any kind of disease." A good number of them (60 out of 90 respondents) is able to describe the reasons for falling sick. A considerable number of them (16 out of 90 respondents) also believe in "attack by ghosts and evil spirits" for causing diseases.

Belief in the existence of super human or super natural power is almost universal. Experiences of certain day-to-day sudden happenings of disease, death and unexplainable have led the Namasudra community into believing in the other than the material visible world, i.e., in the invisible supernatural power. They have established a kind of close relationship between themselves and this power by adjusting themselves to it in two ways, first by controlling or overpowering the spirits by enchanting or practicing some techniques and chanalising the power for good or bad and secondly by offering *puja* or worship to propriate the superhuman power for acquisition of the things or objects desired.

During field investigation the author met an Ojha (traditional medicine man) of Namasudra community who live in Naldungri village in Bongaon Block named Tangra Pagal. He moves from one village to other when the people call in for relief from disease. Tangra Pagal is regarded as Ojha in Namasudra Community. According to him he aquired the power to diagnosis of illness and to give relief from the disease from his guru Late Buddha Pagal of Gopalgunge in Khulna district (at present in Bangladesh). He can cure different types of diseases and according to him he saved the life of Bholanath Biswas of Halencha village from snakebite. The following are some case studies reported regarding their treatment practices of various diseases and ailments:

Case study 1: Durga Biswas, aged 45 years of Bakshipally of Bangaon has been suffering from gastric ulcer and falling of blood from anus since three years. Hearing the name of Tangra Pagal Sri Biswas come to him to cure himself from the disease. After examining the patient Tangra Pagal diagnosed and said that there was an ulcer in the intestine of the patient. The following is the process of treatment of Durga Biswas by Tangra Pagal.

At first the patient is asked to lay down by the side of Sri Sri Harichand temple. The open space infront of the patient is cleared by broomstick and after that the place is plastered with water and cowdung paste. Then Pagal takes a glass of water and puts one tulsi leaf (osimum sanctum and one piece of Durba grass in side the glass of water. He takes tulsi leaf in right hand and puts ' + ' mark on the glass and then dips the leaf and grass in glass of water. He then sprinkles some drop of water on the head of the patient. Then he rubbed the belly region of the patient with that water and the rest portion offered to the patient to drink. After that he is advised to drink the glass of water previously soaked by stool of cockroach (Preiplaneta americana). Then the mixture of extracted juice of Sheuli leaf (Nyctanthes arbortristis-L) mixed in water and lastly mixture of extracted juice of durba grass and water is given to the patient to drink in the name of Sri Sri Harichand Thakur. According to Pagal the patient cured soon day by day.

Case study 2: Kalipada Biswas aged 58 resident of village Kansona has been suffering from bronchitis. He went to Tangra Pagal for his treatment. Pagal gave an amulet to the patient to tie on the upper right arm with a red thread in the name of Sri Sri Harichand Thakur. Before giving the amulet Pagal took a small torn paper on which name of Harichand Thakur was written. Then after rolling that, paper was inserted in the amulet and other end was closed. Then after inserting that paper the open mouth of the amulet was sealed with the help of wax. According to Pagal the patient is somewhat normal.

Case study 3: Netai Biswas of Purana Bongaon aged 35 years has been suffering from harnea for one year. Incidentally at a mela in Satbhai Kalitala he come across Tangra Pagal and he told him about his sufferings. He gave a amulet to the patient to tie on the upper arm with the help of red thread on Wednesday in the name of Sri Sri Harichand Thakur, after finishing the bath, early in the morning. Before handing over amulet to the patient root of Chalta (Dillenia indicus and Dalim or Pune granate (Punia granatum) along with a paper on which name of Harichand Thakur was written inserted into the amulet and the open mouth was sealed with bee wax. Pagal did not claim money for this. On the other hand he advised the patient to offer *puja* in the name of Sri Sri Harichand Thakur after recovery from the suffering.

Case study 4: Shyamali Biswas of Kansona village aged 45 years has been suffering from *Mrigi* or epilepsy for 5 years. She went to Tangra Pagal. Pagal gave the following medicine to Mrs. Biswas. Root of scarlet gourd (Cephalandra indica) is dried in the sun and then it is grinded in the form of powder and mixed with 500 gm of mustard oil and kept in a pot. Then that oil is rubbed on the head of the patient twice daily (in the morning and at night before going to the bed). This process is continued for 3 months and the patient is recovered day by day. According to Mrs. Biswas she was comparatively better.

Case study 5: Binod Bihari Biswas of Kansona village aged

58 years was suffering from jaundice. According to the instruction of Tangra Pagal he was completely cured from this disease. Sri Biswas followed the following process for relief form Jaundice. First of all Binod Biswas took his bath before 5 A.M. The rice soaked in water previous day, mixed with curd (prepared at home) was eaten twice daily in the morning and at night. He continued this treatment for 15 days. Then extracted juice of leaves of pigeon pea (Cajanus indica) mixed with table salt was taken daily early in the morning for seven days. At present he is cured.

The following are the different types of diseases and method of treatment prevalent among the Namasudra Community

Sl.no.	Name of the Disease	Method of treatment
1.	Asthma	Root of parble is put in a amulet and tied on right upper arm with red thread in case of male and on left upper arm in case of female.
2.	Harnea	Pomegranate (Punica granatum) root is inserted in amulet and tied with red thread on the waist of a patient.
3.	High fever	Extracted juice of sheuli leaves (Nyctanthes arbortristis.-L) is given to the patient to drink for consequitive five days.
4.	Epilepsy	Telakuchi (Cephalanda indica) root at first dried and then turned into powder form and then mixed with 500 gms of coconut oil. That oil anointed on head twice daily during morning and night.
5.	Snakebite	The patient is given a mixture of juice of hatisur leaf (Heliotropium indicum) with table salt. After that the doctor is consulted.

6.	Cholera	(a) Curry made by boiled egg with potato and rice is given to the patient to eat. (b) Stool of cockroach (Peripleneta americana) mixed with a glass of water is given to the patient to drink
7.	Small pox	Sandal wood(pterocarpus sankilinus) paste mixed with broken conch-bangle turned into powder form anointed on the effected portion of the patient.
8.	Headache	Grinding black cumin (Jeera) and water mixed in paste form and then applied on the forehead.
9.	Leprosy	At first the patient asked to take his/her bath early in the morning. Then turmeric paste mixed with extracted juice of neem leaf (Melia azadirachta) and that mixture applied on the infected region. Then after one hour that portion is washed by hot water mixed with neem leaf.
10.	Jaundice	a) At first daily bath is to be finished by 5 A.M. then rice mixed with curd and ripe banana is given to the patient. That particular type of diet is to be taken by the patient for consequitive 15 days for better result. b) Extracted juice of Arhar leaf (Cajanu Cajans) is given to the patient to drink for consequitive seven days. That gives better result.
11.	Diabetes	Extracted juice of neem leaf is given to the patient in the morning

after taking bath. Then brinjel and neem leaf mixed and fried with edible oil which is to be eaten during lunch. In the evening extracted juice of Durba grass (Cynodon dactylion) mixed with table salt (NaCl) to be taken. This medicine is to be taken for consequitive 21 days. Then doctor will be consulted. No sweet will be taken.

HEALTH CARE

It is well established that many biosocial variables are involved for survival and well being of a child. To understand biosocial variables in relation to child mortality and survival it is essential to study the effects of different biosocial factors on child survival in a community. In this connection only the last childbirths have been taken into consideration in the present study. The reason for considering the last childbirths is that complete information, regarding that particular delivery is fully available. But if all births are considered, firstly such information will not be available, and secondly there could be many recall lapses. So, for the sake of accuracy of data, observations have been restricted on last childbirths. It has been restricted again for those births, which occurred at any time during the last four years i.e. from 1997 to 2000. In this context a sub-sample has been drawn which consists of 236 live births. Out of which 53 occurred in Purana Bongaon, 124 occurred in Paschim Ramchandrapur and the rest 59 occurred in Kansona village. In the present study altogether 18 biosocial variables have been examined for these three villages. These are: (1) age of respondents; (2) education of respondents; (3) ante-natal check-up of the respondents; (4) iron and folic acid tablets taken by respondents; (5) immunization of respondents; (6) treatment of respondents during pregnancy; (7) place of delivery; (8) delivery attendants; (9)health problem experienced by respondents; (10) treatment of respondents after delivery; (11) breast feeding duration; (12) age of child in which supplementary diet was given: (13) treatment of child; (14)

immunisation of child; 15) family planning method adopted by the respondents ; 16) family planning method adopted by wife/husband ; 17) source of information of family planning; and (18) contraception used/using by mother. In the preceding paragraphs each of the above aspects is described. The observations are based on primary data, which is collected by the present author by interviewing the members of individual families.

Age of the Respondents

In case of the age of respondents at the time of last live birth during last four years (Table 6.1) there exists significant difference between the respondents of Pachim Ramchandrapur and Kansona village. But between Purana Bongaon and Paschim Ramchandrapur and also between Pachim Ramchandrapur and Kansona there exists no significant difference. Though majority of the births occurred among the respondents in 20-24 years and 25-29 years age group in these three villages a considerable per cent of births occurred among higher age group respondents in Paschim Ramchandrapur and Kansona village. In contrast in Purana Bongaon village only a single case of live birth is recorded in 35 years and above age group mothers. This is indicative of consciousness of Purana Bongaon mother regarding the consiquence of health hazards during late age delivery (Table 6.1)

Table 6.1
Age of the respondents

Respond-ents age (in year)	*Village*					
	Purana Bongaon		*Paschim Ramchandrapur*		*Kansona*	
	Numbers	*%*	*Numbers*	*%*	*Numbers*	*%*
20–24	33	62.26	50	40.32	20	33.90
25–29	16	30.19	52	41.94	27	45.76
30–34	3	5.66	10	8.66	7	11.86
35–39	1	1.88	9	7.25	4	6.78
40+	–	–	3	2.42	1	1.69
Total	53	99.99	124	99.99	59	99.99

χ^2 values :

Purana Bonaon (vs) Paschim Ramchandrapur: 8.59 : not significant

Purana Bngaon (vs) Kansona: 10.12 (significant at 0.05 level of probability)

Paschim Ramchandrapur (vs) Kansona : 1.28 : not significant

Education of respondents

Bharati and Ghosh Dastidar (1990) suggest that education of women can improve child bearing and health of entire family. The educated women are more likely to marry at a later age, postpone child bearing, may follow family planning methods and seek consultation with doctor for prenatal care at the time of pregnancy. Regarding education of respondents it is noticed that significant differences exist between the respondents of Purana Bongaon and Paschim Ramchandrapur village, and Paschim Ramchandrapur and Kansona village. But between Paschim Ramchandrapur and Kansona village no significant difference is exist. It can be seen from Table 6.2 that respondents of Purana Bongaon village are better educated than that of village Paschim Ramchandrapur and Kansona. The respondent of Paschim Ramchandrapur in trun is better educated than Kansona. A lower per cent of illiterate respondents are found in village Purana Bongaon (23.41) and Paschim Ramchandrapur (25.81) than that of village Kansona (33.90). It can be recapitulated that infant and toddler mortality are found to be considerably lower in Purana Bongaon and Paschim Ramchandrapur village than that of village Kansona.

Antenatal check-up by respondents

Antenatal care can contribute significantly to the reduction of maternal morbidity as well as mortality because besides offspring medical care it includes advice on the correct diet and provision of necessary medicine to pregnant women (Nair et al., 2000). It is seen from Table 6.3 that more than 90 per cent of the respondents in Purana Bongaon village availed regular medical check-up during pregnancy. The percentage of respondents in Paschim Ramchandrapur and Kansona village in turn are 60.48 and 62.71 respectively in this respect. When the chi² test is performed it is found that both Paschim Ramchandrapur and Kansona villages significantly differ with village Purana Bongaon. But between Paschim Ramchandrapur and Kansona village no significant difference is exist.

Iron and Folic Acid Tablets taken by Respondents

The provision of iron and folic acid tablets acts as prophylactic

Table: 6.2

Education of respondents

Educational status	*Village*					
	Purana Bongaon		*Paschim Ramchandrapur*		*Kansona*	
	Numbers	*%*	*Numbers*	*%*	*Numbers*	*%*
Illiterate	14	26.41	32	25.81	20	33.90
Primary	21	39.62	78	62.90	16	27.12
Secondary and above	18	33.96	14	11.29	23	38.98
Total	53	100.00	124	100.00	59	100.00

χ^2 values :

Purana Bongaon (vs) Paschim Ramchandrapur: 14.16 (significant at 0.05 level of probability)

Purana Bongaon (vs) Kansona: 2.029 : not significant

Paschim Ramchandrapur (vs) Kansona: 26.07 (significant at 0.05 level of probability)

Table: 6.3

Antenatal care of the respondents

Antenatal the respondents during pregnancy	*Village*					
	Purana Bongaon		*Paschim Ramchandrapur*		*Kansona*	
	Numbers	*%*	*Numbers*	*%*	*Numbers*	*%*
Yes	48	90.57	75	60.48	37	62.71
No	5	9.43	49	39.52	22	37.29
Total	53	100.00	124	100.00	59	100.00

χ^2 values :

Purana Bongaon (vs) Paschim Ramchandrapur: 15.84 (significant at 0.05 level of probability)

Purana Bongaon (vs) Kansona: 11.72 (significant at 0.05 level of probability)

Paschim Ramchandrapur (vs) Kansona: 0.08: not significant

against nutritional anaemia among pregnant women, which forms an integral part of the mother child health activities (Nair et al., 2000). It is seen from table 6.4 that there exists no significant difference among the respondents in three villages. It is further noticed that more than 86 per cent of the respondent of village Purana Bongaon and Paschim Ramchandrapur have taken iron and folic acid tablet during pregnancy. while in Kansona village 76.27 per cent mothers have taken this.

Table: 6.4

Iron and folic acid tablets taken by the respondents

Iron and foolic acid tab taken by the respo-dents during Pregnancy	*Village*					
	Purana Bongaon		*Paschim Ramchandrapur*		*Kansona*	
	Numbers	*%*	*Numbers*	*%*	*Numbers*	*%*
Yes	47	88.68	107	86.29	45	76.27
No	6	11.32	17	13.71	14	23.73
Total	53	100.00	124	100.00	59	100.00

χ^2 values :

Purana Bongaon (vs) Paschim Ramchandrapur: 0.19 : not significant
Purana Bongaon (vs) Kansona: 2.93 : not significant
Paschim Ramchandrapur (vs) Kansona: 2.85 : not significant

Immunisation of Expectant Respondents during Pregnancy

Immunization of expectant mother is considered to be an important aspect of health care of women during pregnancy. It is noticed from Table 6.5 that more than 98 per cent respondents in Purana Bongaon and 96 per cent in Paschim Ramchandrapur village have taken tetanus injection during pregnancy. While in Kansona village 89.93 respondents are found who have taken this. These indicate that respondents in all the villages are well aware of the benefit of this immunisation. When the chi^2 test is applied it is found that no such significant differences exist among the respondents of these three villages.

Treatment of Respondents during Pregnancy

It is evident from Table 6.6 that more than 92 per cent respondents in Purana Bongaon and 86 per cent in Kansona preferred treatment by medical persons during pregnancy. In contrast 65.52 per cent respondents in Paschim Ramchandrapur village preferred treatment by medical persons. Side by side, only 7.51 per cent respondents in Purana Bongaon preferred treatment by non-medical persons, while 35.48 per cent respondents in Paschim Ramchandrapur village have preferred this treatment. From the results of chi² test it appears that there is significant difference among the respondents between Purana Bongaon and Paschim Ramchandrapur as well as between Paschim Ramchandrapur and Kansona in this respect.

Place of Delivery

In respect of place of delivery two sub-variables namely, delivery at hospital or nursing home and delivery at home, have been considered. It is seen from Table 6.7 that more than 47 per cent respondents in Purana Bongaon have opted for hospital or nursing home delivery, whereas more than 72 per cent respondents of Paschim Ramchandrapur and 80 per cent respondents of Kansona have opted for delivery at home. Table 6.7 indicates that in respect of place of delivery there is significant difference among the respondents between Purana Bongaon and Paschim Ramchandrapur village, and Purana Bongaon and Kansona village.

Table : 6.5

Tetanus injections taken by the respondents

Titenus injections taken by the respondents during pregnancy	*Village*					
	Purana Bongaon		*Paschim Ramchandrapur*		*Kansona*	
	Numbers	*%*	*Numbers*	*%*	*Numbers*	*%*
Yes	52	98.11	119	95.97	53	89.83
No	1	1.89	5	4.03	6	10.17
Total	53	100.00	124	100.00	59	100.00

χ^2 values :

Purana Bongaon (vs) Paschim Ramchandrapur : 0.52 : not significant

Purana Bongaon (vs) Kansona: 3.28 : not significant

Paschim Ramchandrapur (vs) Kansona: 2.673 : not significant

Table: 6.6

Treatment of respondents during pregnancy in three villages

Treatment of respondents during pregnancy	*Village*					
	Purana Bongaon		*Paschim Ramchandrapur*		*Kansona*	
	Numbers	*%*	*Numbers*	*%*	*Numbers*	*%*
Medical	49	92.49	80	65.52	51	86.44
Non Medical	4	7.51	44	35.48	8	13.56
Total	53	100.00	124	100.00	59	100.00

χ^2 values :

Purana Bongaon (vs) Paschim Ramchandrapur: 14.65
(significant at 0.05 level of probability)

Purana Bongaon (vs) Kansona: 1.05: not significant

Paschim Ramchandrapur (vs) Kansona: 9.43
(significant at 0.05 level of probability)

Table: 6.7

Place of delivery of the respondents

Place of delivery	*Village*					
	Purana Bongaon		*Paschim Ramchandrapur*		*Kansona*	
	Numbers	*%*	*Numbers*	*%*	*Numbers*	*%*
Hospital / Nursing Home	25	47.17	34	27.41	11	18.64
Home	28	52.83	90	72.58	48	81.36
Total	53	100.00	124	100.00	59	100.00

χ^2 values :

Purana Bongaon (vs) Paschim Ramchandrapur : 6.51
(significant at 0.05 level of probability)

Purana Bongaon (vs) Kansona: 10.40
(significant at 0.05 level of probability)

Paschim Ramchandrapur (vs) Kansona: 1.65: not significant

But between Paschim Ramchandrapur and Kansona village there exists no significant difference in this respect.

Delivery Attendant

Like the earlier variable in this case also significant differences exist amont the respondents of Purana Bongaon and Paschim Ramchandrapur village, and Purana Bongaon and Kansona village, while between Paschim Ramchandrapur and Kansona village no significant difference is noticed. It can be seen from Table 6.8 that more than 73 per cent deliveries in Paschim Ramchandrapur and 81 per cent deliveries in Kansona have been attended by untrained Dai's, while in Purana Bongaon village near about 53 per cent deliveries are attended by untrained Dai's. However, a good per cent of deliveries (47.17) in Purana Bongaon village are found to be attended by the Doctor or Nurses.

Health Problem experienced by Respondents after First Week of Delivery

It is seen from Table 6.9 that 47.17 per cent of the respondents in Purana Bongaon village have experienced health problem after first week of delivery, while 25.80 per cent respondents in Paschim Ramchandrapur and 27.12 per cent respondents in Kansona have experienced health problem after first week of delivery. When the chi^2 test is performed it is found that there is significant difference among the respondents between Purana Bongaon and Paschim Ramchandrapur village and between Purana Bongaon and Kansona village, while between Paschim Ramchandrapur and Kansona village no significant difference is noticed.

Treatment of Respondents after Delivery

In respect of treatment of respondents after delivery it is found that a higher per cent of respondents in Purana Bongaon village (45.28) have preferred medical treatment than that of Paschim Ramchandrapur (24.19) and Kansona village (23.73). However, in Paschim Ramchandrapur and Kansona village more than 75 per cent respondents have been found to prefer non-medical treatment. Table 6.10 indicates that there are significant differences among the respondents between Purana Bongaon and Paschim

Ramchandrapur village, and Purana Bongaon and Kansona village, But between Paschim Ramchandrapur and Kansona there exist no significant difference.

Table: 6.8

Delivery attendants of the respondents

Delivery of respondents	*Village*					
	Purana Bongaon		*Paschim Ramchandrapur*		*Kansona*	
	Numbers	*%*	*Numbers*	*%*	*Numbers*	*%*
Doctor /Nurse	25	47.17	33	26.61	11	18.64
Untrained Dai	28	52.83	91	73.38	48	81.36
Total	53	100.00	124	99.99	59	100.00

χ^2 values :

Purana Bongaon (vs) Paschim Ramchandrapur : 7.12
(significant at 0.05 level of probability)

Purana Bongaon (vs) Kansona: 10.40
(significant at 0.05 level of probability)

Paschim Ramchandrapur (vs) Kansona: 1.39: not significant

Table: 6.9

Health problem experienced by the respondents

Health problem experieced after frist week of delivery	*Village*					
	Purana Bongaon		*Paschim Ramchandrapur*		*Kansona*	
	Numbers	*%*	*Numbers*	*%*	*Numbers*	*%*
Yes	25	47.17	32	25.80	16	27.12
No	28	52.83	92	74.19	43	72.88
Total	53	100.00	124	99.99	59	100.00

χ^2 values :

Purana Bongaon (vs) Paschim Ramchandrapur: 7.75
(significant at 0.05 level of probability)

Purana Bongaon (vs) Kansona : 4.81
(significant at 0.05 level of probability)

Paschim Ramchandrapur (vs) Kansona: 0.03: not significant

Table: 6.10

Treatment of the respondents after delivery

Treatment of respondents after delivery	*Village*					
	Purana Bongaon		*Paschim Ramchandrapur*		*Kansona*	
	Numbers	*%*	*Numbers*	*%*	*Numbers*	*%*
Medical	24	45.28	30	24.19	14	23.73
Non-Medical	29	54.72	94	75.81	45	76.27
Total	53	100.00	124	100.00	59	100.00

χ^2 values :

Purana Bongaon (vs) Paschim Ramchandrapur : 7.79
(significant at 0.05 level of probability)

Purana Bongaon (vs) Kansona: 5.76
(significant at 0.05 level of probability)

Paschim Ramchandrapur (vs) Kansona : 0.00: not significant

Table: 6.11

Breast feeding duration by the respondents

Duration of breast feeding (in years)	*Village*					
	Purana Bongaon		*Paschim Ramchandrapur*		*Kansona*	
	Numbers	*%*	*Numbers*	*%*	*Numbers*	*%*
< 1	19	35.85	38	30.64	10	16.95
1 – 2	20	37.73	31	25.00	33	55.93
2 +	14	26.41	55	44.35	16	27.12
Total	53	99.99	124	99.99	59	100.00

χ^2 values :

Purana Bongaon (vs) Paschim Ramchandrapur: 5.47
: not significant

Purana Bongaon (vs) Kansona : 5.81
: not significant

Paschim Ramchandrapur (vs) Kansona: 19.85
(significant at 0.05 level of probability)

Breast Feeding Duration

Breast feeding has important health advantages for infants and children. Research based on data from diverse sources provides convincing evidence of the positive effects of breast feeding and long birth intervals on survival of the children (Cleland and Sathar, 1984). It reveals from Table 6.11 that 44.35 per cent of the respondents in Paschim Ramchandrapur have breast feeded their babies for more than two years, whereas in Purana Bongaon and Kansona village this percentage value is found to be 26.41 and 27.12 respectively. In the category of below 1 years breast feeding duration more than 30 per cent respondents are found in Purana Bongaon and Paschim Ramchandrapur village. However, when chi^2 test is performed it is seen that there is significant difference among the respondents between Paschim Ramchandrapur and Kansona village. But between Purana Bongaon and Paschim Ramchandrapur, and Puran Bongaon and Kansona no significant difference is noticed.

Age of Children at First Supplementary Diet given

It can be seen from Table 6.12 that about 60 per cent of the children of the respondents in Kansona village taken their first supplementary diet during their 7-8 months of age. Side by side this percentage is 38.71 and 32.07 in Paschim Ramchandrapur and Purana Bongaon respectively in this age group. Though more than 30 per cent of the children in these two villages have taken their first supplementary diet during 6 months of age in Kansona only 18.64 per cent children are reported in this category. In application of chitest it is found that there is significant difference among the children between village Purana Bongaon and Kansona but in other two cases no significant difference is noticed.

Treatment of Child

In respect of treatment of child (medical or non-medical) significant differences exist among the children of the respondents of Purana Bongaon and Pashim Ramchandrapur village and Paschim Ramchandrapur and Kansona village, whereas between Purana Bogaon and Kansona no significant difference is noticed. It is observed that more than 80 per cent of the children of the respondents in Purana Bongaon and Kansona availed treatment by medical doctors, whereas 54 per cent of the children in Paschim Ramchandrapur availed this. Thus, treatment by non-medical doctor is comparatively high in Paschim Ramchandrapur (45.96) than that of Purana Bonaon (18.86) and Kansona (15.25) village (Table 6.13).

Table: 6.12

Age of child in which first supplementary diet was given by the respondents

Age of child at the first supplementary diet was given (in month)	*Village*					
	Purana Bongaon		*Paschim Ramchandrapur*		*Kansona*	
	Numbers	*%*	*Numbers*	*%*	*Numbers*	*%*
6	18	33.96	40	32.25	11	18.64
7-8	17	32.07	48	38.71	33	55.93
9+	18	33.96	36	29.03	15	25.42
Total	53	99.99	124	99.99	59	99.99

χ^2 values :

Purana Bongaon (vs) Paschim Ramchandrapur : 0.77 : not significant

Purana Bongaon (vs) Kansona : 6.78 (significant at 0.05 level of probability)

Paschim Ramchandrapur (vs) Kansona: 5.52 : not significant

Table: 6.13

Treatment of child of the respondents

Treatment of child	*Village*					
	Purana Bongaon		*Paschim Ramchandrapur*		*Kansona*	
	Numbers	*%*	*Numbers*	*%*	*Numbers*	*%*
Medical	43	1.13	67	54.03	50	84.75
Non-medical	10	18.86	57	45.96	9	15.25
Total	53	99.99	124	99.99	59	100.00

χ^2 values :

Purana Bongaon (vs) Paschim Ramchandrapur : 11.60 (significant at 0.05 level of probability)

Purana Bongaon (vs) Kansona : 0.43 : not significant

Paschim Ramchandrapur (vs) Kansona : 16.35 (significant at 0.05 level of probability)

Table: 6.14

Immunisation of child of the respondents

Immunisation of Child	*Village*					
	Purana Bongaon		*Paschim Ramchandrapur*		*Kansona*	
	Numbers	*%*	*Numbers*	*%*	*Numbers*	*%*
Completed	25	47.17	32	25.80	14	23.73
Partly completed	23	43.40	75	60.48	36	61.02
Not taken	5	9.43	17	13.71	9	15.25
Total	53	100.00	124	99.99	59	100.00

χ^2 values :

Purana Bongaon (vs) Paschim Ramchandrapur : 7.74
(significant at 0.05 level of probability)

Purana Bongaon (vs) Kansona: 6.78
(significant at 0.05 level of probability)

Paschim Ramchandrapur (vs) Kansona : 0.74 : not significant

Immunisation of Child

Immunisation status of the child of the respondents is shown in Table 6.14 according to villages. More than 47 per cent of the children in Purana Bongaon have completed their immunisation, while in Paschim Ramchandrapur and Kansona 25.8 and 23.73 per cent of the children have completed immunisation. A high per cent of the children have partly completed immunisation in all three villages. However, this percentage is much higher is Paschim Ramchandrapur (60.48) and Kansona (61.02) village than that of Purana Bongaon (43.40) village. When Chi² test is performed it is seen that there is significant difference among the child of the respondents of Purana Bongaon and Paschim Ramchandrapur, and Purana Bongaon and Kansona village. But between Paschim Ramchandrapur and Kansona no significant difference is noticed in this respect.

In order to collect necessary information on contraception 236 mothers were randomly choosen, which consists of 53, 124 and 59 mothers for village Purana Bongaon, Paschim Ramchandrapur and Kansona respectively.

Family Planning Method adopted by Respondents

It reveals from Table 6.15 that only 7.25 per cent of the respondents in Paschim Ramchandrapur have adopted family planning methods, whereas in other two villages this value is found to be quite encouraging. In Purana Bongaon and Kansona village more than one fourth of the respondents have adopted family planning methods. Respondents of Purana Bongaon and Paschim Ramchandrapur, and Paschim Ramchandrapur and Kansona differ significantly. While between Purana Bongaon and Kansona there is no significant difference in this respect.

Who initiated Family Planning?

It is seen from Table 6.16 that the wives are found to initiate family planning in these villages. Percentage of this is found to be highest in Paschim Ramchandrapur (83.33) and lowest in Purana Bongaon (58.33) village while village Kansona (66.66) stands in between in this respect. However, in Purana Bongaon village a good per cent of husband (41.67) are found who initiated family planning. When the chi^2 test is performed it is found that there exists no significant difference among the respondents in these three villages.

Source of Information Regarding Family Planning

It can be seen from Table 6.17 that more than 70 per cent respondents in Paschim Ramchandrapur received necessary information of family planning from their neighbours, friends and relatives. The percentage of which is found to be 50.94 in Purana Bongaon and 59.32 in Kansona. However, a good per cent of respondent in Purana Bongaon (49.05) and Kansona (40.68) are found to receive necessary information on family planning from the health workers. In this respect the respoundents of Purana Bongaon and Paschim Ramchandrapur differ significantly, whereas in other cases no significant difference is noticed.

Table: 6.15

Adoption of family planning by the respondents

Family Planning method adopted	Village.					
	Purana Bongaon		Paschim Ramchandrapur		Kansona	
	Numbers	%	Numbers	%	Numbers	%
Yes	15	28.30	9	7.25	15	25.42
No	38	71.70	115	92.74	44	74.58
Total	53	100.00	124	99.99	59	100.00

χ^2 values :

Purana Bongaon (vs) Paschim Ramchandrapur :14.03

(significant at 0.05 level of probability)

Purana Bongaon (vs) Kansona : 0.12 : not significant

Paschim Ramchandrapur (vs) Kansona : 11.59

(significant at 0.05 level of probability)

Table: 6.16

Family Planning method adopted by whom

Family Planning method adopted by	Village					
	Purana Bongaon		Paschim Ramchandrapur		Kansona	
	Numbers	%	Numbers	%	Numbers	%
Husband	5	41.67	1	16.66	2	33.33
Wife	7	58.33	5	83.33	4	66.66
Total	12*	100.00	6**	99.99	6***	99.99

* data from 3 respondents could not be collected

** data from 3 respondents could not be collected

*** data from 9 respondents could not be collected

χ^2 values :

Purana Bongaon (vs) Paschim Ramchandrapur:1.12 : not significant

Purana Bongaon (vs) Kansona: 0.11 : not significant

Paschim Ramchandrapur (vs) Kansona : 0.44 : not significant

Table: 6.17

Source of information regarding Family planning methods

Source of information	*Village*					
	Purana Bongaon		*Paschim Ramchandrapur*		*Kansona*	
	Numbers	*%*	*Numbers*	*%*	*Numbers*	*%*
ANM [Health worker]	26	49.05	37	29.84	24	40.68
Neighbour / Friend/Relatives	27	50.94	87	70.16	35	59.32
Total	53	99.99	124	100.00	59	100.00

χ^2 values :

Purana Bongaon (vs) Paschim Ramchandrapur: 5.97 (significant at 0.05 level of probability)

Purana Bongaon (vs) Kansona : 0.79 : not significant

Paschim Ramchandrapur (vs) Kansona : 3.07 : not significant

Contraception used by the Respondents

In respect of contraception used by the respondents it is found from the Table 6.18 that most of them used oral pill to restrict their pregnancy. This percentage is 58.49, 72.58 and 72.88 in Purana Bongaon, Paschim Ramchandrapur and Kansona villages respectively. However, a good per cent of husband (33.96) is found in Purana Bongaon to use condom as contraceptive. This percentage is moderate in Paschim Ramchandrapur (23.39) and low (16.95) in Kansona village. A few number of them also used other methods in this respect. When chi² test is performed it is found that there exists no significant difference among the respondents residing in these three villages.

Taking into consideration all these variables it is found from Table 6.19 that the respondents of Purana Bongaon differ from the respondents of Paschim Ramchandrapur in 11 variables out of 18 and from Kansona in 8 out of 18 variables, whereas between Paschim Ramchandrapur and Kansona the significant differences have been noticed in 5 out of 18 variables.

Table : 6.18

Contraception used / using by the couples

Contraception used/using	*Village*					
	Purana Bongaon		*Paschim Ramchandrapur*		*Kansona*	
	Numbers	*%*	*Numbers*	*%*	*Numbers*	*%*
Condom	18	33.96	29	23.39	10	16.95
Oral pill	31	58.49	90	72.58	43	72.88
Others	4	7.55	5	4.03	6	10.17
Total	53	100.00	124	100.00	59	100.00

χ^2 values :

Purana Bongaon (vs) Paschim Ramchandrapur: 3.54 : not significant

Purana Bongaon (vs) Kansona: 4.32 : not significant

Paschim Ramchandrapur (vs) Kansona : 3.28 : not significant

Table : 6.19

Biosocial factors in relation to health care practices

Sl.no	*Biosocial factors*	*Village*		
		Purana Bangaon Vs Paschim Ramchandrapur	*Purana Bangaon Vs Kansona*	*Paschim Ramchandrapur Vs Kansona*
1	Age of mother	–	+	–
2	Education of mother	+	–	+
3	Antenatal check–up by mother	+	+	–
4	Iron and folic acid tablets taken by mother	–	–	–
5	Immunization of expectant mother during pregnancy	–	–	–
6	Treatment of mother during pregnancy	+	–	+
7	Place of delivery	+	+	–
8	Delivery attendant	+	+	–
9	Health problem experienced by mother after delivery	+	+	–
10	Treatment of mother after Delivery	+	+	–

Sl.no	Biosocial factors	Village		
		Purana Bangaon Vs Paschim Ramchandrapur	Purana Bangaon Vs Kansona	Paschim Ramchandrapur Vs Kansona
11	Breast–feeding duration	–	–	+
12	Age of child in which first supplementary diet was given	–	+	–
13	Treatment of child	+	–	+
14	Immunization of child	+	+	–
15	Family planning method adopted by mother	+	–	+
16	Who initiated family planning?	–	–	–
17	Source of information regarding family planning	+	–	–
18	Contraception used / using by the couples	–	–	–

Note : + = Significant
– = Non Significant

Family Planning and Fertility:

In order to collect necessary information on family planning and fertility, average live births of the adopters and non-adopters (family planning methods) were calculated. It is seen from Table 6.20 that average live births is comparatively low among the adopters of family planning methods in all the villages, which again is more marked in Purana Bongaon and Paschim Ramchandra village.

Table: 6.20
Family planning methods and fertility

Family planning methods	Village					
	Purana Bongaon		Paschim Ramchandrapur		Kansona	
	No.	Average	No.	Average	No.	Average
Adopted	15	2.79	9	3.51	15	3.78
Non adopted	38	3.58	115	3.89	44	4.21

7

DISCUSSION AND CONCLUSION

Discussion

In the present work general demographic features deal with size and composition of family, age-sex composition and civil condition, educational and occupational status of the spouses in Purana Bongaon, Paschim Ramchandrapur and Kansona village.

Males are found to be more in number than the females, when the total population according to age and sex is taken into consideration. Of the total population 31.02 per cent males and 34.30 per cent females fall in the age group 0-14 years, while in 15-49 years age group 56.01 per cent males and 52.92 percent females are found. The rest of the population fall in 50 years and above age group. When the distribution of the Namasudra population according to villages is examined it is found that a significant excess of males relative to females is observed in each of the villages. Higher number of males than that of the females is noticed in Purana Bongaon in 20-24 years and 25-29 years age group. But in 40-44 years age group a reverse trend is perceptible. There is a considerable increase of individuals from 0-4 years to 5-9 years age group in both the sexes in Paschim Ramchandrapur village. In 10-14 years and 25-29 years age group considerably higher per cent of females are noticed than the males, while in 20-24 years age group a reverse trend is evident in this village. It appears in case of village Kansona that there is a significant increase in number of individuals from 0-4 years to 5-9 years age group in both the sexes, and from 5-9 years age group onwards a gradual decrease in the number of individuals in evident. Population pyramid of the Namasudra residing in Purana Bongaon and Paschim Ramchandrapur village exhibits a progressive type population growth in the village, while in village Kansona, a constriction at the base of the population pyramid, suggests a recent fertility decline, or increased infant mortality. Population pyramid characterising with progressive type population growth is seen among the Raj Gond of Sagar district, Madhya Pradesh (Tiwari *et al.,* 2002), War Khasi of Meghalaya (Khongsdier, 1991), Garo of Shillong (Adak, 1993), Khamti of Arunachal Pradesh (Chowdhury *et al.,* 1994) and others. Side by side, population pyramid characterising with recent fertility decline or increased infant mortality is seen among the Hajong of Meghalaya (Adak *et al.,* 1999), Namasudra of Midnapur, West Bengal (Mukhopadhay, 1981), Ladiya of Sagar district, Madhya Pradesh (Adak and Gharami, 2001) Naik Gond of Chandrapur district, Maharastra (Rao, 1989) and others. However, When the sex-ratio in pre-reproductive (0-14 years), reproductive (15-49 years) and post-reproductive (50+ years) age groups for the Namasudra residing in studied villages are taken into consideration, it is seen that in all these categories the males are always found to be excess over females, which is clearly reflected in the sex-ratio values. Exceptions in this case are reflected in pre-reproductive age group in Paschim Ramchandrapur and Kansona village. Higher number of males than the females in these three age groups is also found among the Ladiya of Sagar district, Madhya Pradesh (Adak and Gharami, 2001).

Nuclear type of families is found in majority among the Namasudra residing in these villages. Side by side, medium type of families is found to be more frequent among them. When the marital status of this population is taken into consideration it is noticed that all the males below 19 years of age in Purana Bongaon and Kansona, and all the males below 15 years of age in Paschim Ramchandrapur are unmarried. Side by side, all the females below 15 years of age are unmarried. A good number of widows are recorded in Paschim

Ramchandrapur. But except a single case of female divorcee in Paschim Ramchandrapur no case of divorcee is found in these villages. It is interesting to note that near about one fourth of the husbands are illiterate among the Namasudra residing in three villages. In turn 30.55 percent women in Paschim Ramchandrapur, 34.91 percent women in Purana Bongaon and 42.91 percent women in Kansona village are found to be illiterate. Thus the female section in study population exhibits a high percentage of illiteracy. It is well established that infant mortality rate is influenced by the mother's educational level. Inverse relationship between infant mortality and mother's educational level has also been revealed by many studies (Stockwell and Hutchinson, 1975; Knowles and Anker, 1975; Kelley, 1976; Butz and Devanzo, 1978). Ahigh level of illiteracy among the study population indicates a possibility of high infant mortality rate among them.

The mean number of live births among the Namasudra is found to be 3.49, which is comparatively higher than the Namasudra (3.06) of Balaramchak, Midnapore district, West Bengal (Mukhopadhyay, 1981). But it is almost equal to the Ladiya of Madhya Pradesh (Adak and Gharami, 2001), Raj Gond of Madhya Pradesh (Tiwari *et al.,* 2002) and Khamti of Arunchal Pradesh (Chowdhury *et. al.,* 1994) but it is comparatively lower than that of the Hajong of Meghalaya (Adak *et al.*, 1999). When the village-wise number of live births is considered for three villages it is found that Purana Bongaon shows the lowest average of live births (3.08) and Kansona shows the highest (3.71), whereas Paschim Ramchandrapur stands in between (3.54) in this respect. However, when the numbers of married women of active reproductive span (i.e., 15-49 years) and surviving sibship size are taken into consideration for three villages it is seen that mean number of surviving children increases from Purana Bongaon (2.37) to Kansona (2.72) through Paschim Ramchandrapur (2.63), which is indicative of fertility increment with the increment in geographic distance from urban centre. A similar trend is perceptible when percent of infant mortality is taken into consideration in three locations. Infant mortality is found to be lowest in Purana Bongaon (3.85 %) and highest in Kansona (6.30%), while in Paschim Ramchandrapur an intermediate rate (4.83%) is recorded. The incidence of infant mortality is, however, much higher in Kansona than that of Purana Bongaon and Paschim Ramchandrapur. When the rate of infant mortality is calculated it is found that this rate is 50.75 per 1000 live births among the Namasudra which is comparatively lower than West Bengal State level date (i.e. 53 per 1000 live births). But the same is much lower than the Raj Gond (Tiwari *et al.* 2002), and Ladiya (Adak, 2001) of Madhya Pradesh, Khamti of Arunachal Pradesh (Chowdhury *et al.* 1994) and Hajong of Meghalaya (Adak *et al.* 1999). Infant mortality is used as a reliable and sensitive indicator of health status in any community. Lower incidence of infant mortality among the study population in Purana Bongaon is indicative of better health standard of the community and higher incidence of infant mortality in Kansona is indicative of poor health standard of the community. Whereas, the Namasudra of Paschim Ramchandrapur stands in between in this respect, among whom also a better standard of health is indicative.

It is well established that availability of health care facilities diminishes with the geographic distances of the locations increases from the nearest urban centre. It can be recapitulated that the three villages under study are located in three different geographic locations from the Block Headquarter. Is there exist considerable differences in terms of health care practices among the Namasudra residing in three different location? Keeping this in view a further probe has been made into matter considering 18 health related variables. In this connection only the cases of last child births, which took place during last four years were taken into consideration. The reason behind this is that complete information regarding that particular delivery, was fully available. In case of earlier births such detailed information are not generally available, and secondly there are strong possibility of many recall lapses.

Taking into consideration all the variables it is found that the respondents of Purana Bongaon differ from the respondents of Paschim Ramchandrapur in 11 variables out of 18 and from Kansona in 8 out of 18 variables, whereas between Paschim Ramchandrapur and Kansona significant differences have been noticed in 5 out of 18 variables. It reveals that the Namasudra residing (*i.e.,* of Purana Bongaon) nearer to sub-divisional health centre, which is located in block head quarter town Bongaon, are in better position of health than that of the Namasudra of other two locations. Side by side, Namasudra of Paschim Ramchandrapur, which is located nearer to Bongaon town than Kansona, is found in better position of health than that of Kansona in this respect. It appears that the Namasudra of Purana Bongaon largely depend on modern medical treatment like immunisation of child, delivery in hospital or nursing home rather than at home, treatment by professional medical doctors rather than by the quacks. Besides, it is also noticed that a good number of couple among them have adopted family planning method. Side by side, the Namasudra of Paschim Ramchandrapur are in better position in respect of place of delivery, medical check-up of mother during pregnancy and treatment of the child than the Namasudra of Kansona. Consequently both infant and toddler mortality are found to be lowest among the Namasudra of Purana Bongaon and highest in Kansona, whereas the Namasudra of Paschim Ramchandrapur stands in between in this respect.

Thus in fine it can be said that due to the nearness of the urban centre the Namasudra of Purana Bongaon certainly enjoy better medical and public health facilities than their counterparts in other two locations. Side by side, due to the relative proximity of the village Paschim Ramchandrapur to the urban centre, the Namasudra in this location enjoy comparatively better medical facilities than the Namasudra of Kansona village, which is located at a far distance from sub-divisional health centre located in Bongaon town. This buttressed the incidence of infant and toddler mortality among the study population residing in three different locations, which is also indicative of better health consciousness among the Namasudra of Purana Bongaon than other two villages and comparatively less consciousness of health among the Namasudra of Kansona than other two villages.

Conclusion

Health seeking is an important factor in health management, but in a country like India, where most of health schemes are centralised, this is often ignored while considering for providing health facilities to the people. The decision makers in the health sector are recognising the need for understanding the health seeking behaviour and perception of the communities and their acceptance and usage of traditional and modern methods, as also the perception of the community regarding the service delivery. This is relevant especially to the communities belong to weaker sections.

Health care is a high priority in all developing countries and is a constitutional right in a number of them. Over the past five years India's national policies have shifted sharply from expansion of facilities for hospital-based care towards extension of rudimentary health services to the underserved (particularly rural) populations.

It is observed that the public health centres in our country are essentially curative, capital intensive and are oriented towards the rich in urban areas. The people in urban areas generally get the lion's share of medical resources. While assessing their impact in rural areas it is necessary to thoroughly examine if the public health centres are well equipped in terms of professional expertise and staff members. However, the fact remains that though the public health facilities are to paly dominant role in the lives of the patients belonging to the rural areas, but their performances have not been perfect and adequate in many areas. Therefore, there is urgent need to update our present knowledge about health status and health care practices among various weaker sections in our country.

Indian rural economy is largely based on agriculture, but the main economic source, the land is generally owned by several middle and hgher-class caste groups. The scheduled castes, scheduled tribes and other backward castes from the economically weaker sections in the society. In West Bengal in general, and North Twenty Four Parganas district in particular the scheduled caste groups lead a precarious life and their health status too is generally poor.

In the present work, reproductive behaviour and health care practices have been studied among the Namasudra scheduled caste population of West Bengal.

They are mostly concentrated in North Twenty Four Parganas

district in the State. However, their highest concentration is found in North Twenty Four Parganas district. Again in North Twenty Four Parganas, their highest concentration is found in Bongaon block. The total population of Namasudra in West Bengal according to 1981 census was 1,692,238. A considerable number of them (i.e., 18.15%) are residing in urban area. The literacy rate of the Namasudra according to 1981 census was 35.87 % (the male and female literacy was 45.71 and 25.09 respectively). The area selected for the present study is Bongaon, a Namasudra predominant block in North Twenty Four Parganas district of West Bengal. Namasudra are not an occupational caste. They are found in various occupations as cultivators, fishermen, boatmen, carpenters etc. They are regarded as untouchables by the higher castes of Bengal, and a generation ago was known by the name *Chandals*. Numerically they are second major scheduled caste of West Bengal.

For collection of data random sample technique was employed. At the first stage North Twenty Four Parganas district of West Bengal was purposively selected to ensure maximum coverage of Namasudra community and to minimise the cost and time involved in the survey and to facilitate maximum utilisation of the time available for research. Out of 22 Community Development Blocks of North Twenty Four Parganas district further Bongaon Block was purposively selected because of intensive coverage of Namasudra population in this blick. The data of the present study were collected from three villages located in three different locations in Bongaon block, which are as follows:

Village – I : Purana Bongaon – located nearest to the sub-divisional health centre (3 km far);

Village – II : Paschim Ramchandrapur – located far from the sub-divisional health centre (7 km far) and

Village – III : Kansona – located at a location farthest (12 km.) from the sub-divisional health centre.

In the present study altogether 876 couples were interviewed. Data were collected from above selected villages using schedules/ qustionnaries and case study.

It appears from the age sex composition of the Namasudra that the males are numerically more than the females in all the three locations. Sex ratio values of the study population in Purana Bongaon. Paschim Ramchandrapur and Kansona are found to be 89.12, 92.48 and 94.24 respectively. About 33 per cent of the total population is in the pre-reproductive age group (0-14 years), whereas in reproductive (15-49 years) and post-reproductive age group (50 years and above) 53 percent and 13 per cent of the total population are found in these three villages. In Purana Bongaon the husbands are found to be engaged mailnly in daily labour, rickshaw pulling and business, while in Paschim Ramchandrapur they are found to be engaged mainly in daily labour and different kind of business. But in Kansona the husbands are mainly engaged in their own agriculture and agricultural labour. Majority of the wives in these three villages are found to be housewife excepting village Purana Bongaon where most of them are engaged in bidi binding job. When the educational status of the couples is taken into consideration it is found that about 24 per cent of the husbands and 32 per cent of the wives are illiterate, excepting village Kansona where 42 per cent wives are found to be illiterate.

In order to collect necessary information on reproductive performance altogether 876 couples (202 couples from Purana Bongaon, 426 couples from Paschim Ramchandrapur, and 248 couples from Kansona) were interviewed by drawing estended genealogies, maintaining several suitable crosschecks. Knowledgeable and experienced persons were also extensively interviewed to adopt case study methods.

Mean live births among the Namasudra is found to be 3.49. This ranges between 3.08 to 3.71 in three locations, which is lowest in Purana Bongaon (*i.e.*, 3.08) and highest in Kansona (*i.e.*, 3.71) and Paschim Ramchandrapur village stands in between (*i.e.*, 3.54). Thus, the level of fertility increases among the Namasudra as the geographic distance of their location increases from the sub-divisional health centre. This is true in case of mortality rate also. Rate of infant (0-1 year) and toddler mortality (1-4 years) is found to be 50.75 and 18.01 respectively per 1000 live births among the Namasudra. However, when the same is calculated in three different locations it is found to be lowest in Purana Bongaon (38.52 per 1000 live births) and highest in Kansona village (62.97 per 1000 live births). However, in Paschim Ramchandrapur an intermediate rate (48.34 per 1000 live births) is obtained. In case of toddler mortality also (1-4 years) a similar trend is noticed. Rate of toddler mortality is found to be lowest in Purna Bongaon (11.23 per 1000 live births) and highest in Kansona (31.49 per 1000 live births). However, the village Paschim Ramchandrapur stands in between in this respect. Rate of toddler mortality is found to be 12.58 per 1000 live births in this village. When the rates of infant mortality among the Namasudra is compared with the national level data it is found that this rate is considerable lower among them than our national average. This is true for the Namasudra residing in three different locations. However, when the infant mortality rates of the study population is compared with the State level data it is noticed that this is considerabley lower among the Namasudra residing in Purana Bongaon and Paschim Ramchandrapur but considerably higher in Kansona than that of the West Bengal state level data (*i.e.,* 53 per 1000 live births). Infant mortality rate is always used as a reliable and sensitive indicator of health status in a community. Low rate of infant mortality among the Namasudra of Purana Bongaon reflects a better standard of health among them. Side by side, its high rate in Kansona reflects a poor standard of health among the study population. However, Namasudra of Paschim Ramchandrapur stands in between in this respect.

For a further probe into this matter immunisation and childcare, prenatal and postnatal care of the mothers and contraception methods followed by this population are examined. In this connection only the last child birth, which took place during last four years were taken into consideration. The reason for considering the last childbirths that complete information, regarding that particular delivery, was fully available. In case of earlier births such detailed information are not generally available, and secondly there are strong possibility of many recall lapses.

Taking into consideration all the variables it is found that in respect of different variables there exist considerable differences among the Namasudra residing in three different locations. And it holds good that the Namasudra residing nearer to sub-divisional health centre (i.e., in Purana Bongaon) are in better position of health than that of the Namasudra of other two locations. Side by side, Namasudra of Paschim Ramchandrapur is in better position than that of the Kansona in this respect. It is found that the Namasudra of Purana Bongaon largely depend on modern medical treatment like immunisation of child, delivery in health centre rather than at home, treatment by professional medical doctors rather than by the quacks and have better sense of personal hygience. Besides it is also noticed that a good number of couples among them have adopted family planning method. Side by side, the Namasudra of Paschim Ramchandrapur is in better position in respect of place of delivery, medical check-up of mother during pregnancy and treatment of the child than the Namasudra of Kansona. Consequently, both infant and toddler mortality rates among the Namasudra are lowest in Purana Bongaon and highest in Kansona and the Namasudra of Paschim Ramchandrapur stands in between. It can be recapitulated that the village Purana Bongaon is located nearer to the block headquarter, where the sub-divisional health centre is located and the village Kansona is located far apart from the sub-divisional health centre. The village Paschim Ramchandrapur, however, located in-between these two villages. Due to the nearness of the urban centre the Namasudra of Purana Bongaon certainly enjoy better medical and public health facilities than their counterparts in other two locations. Side by side, due to the relative proximity of the village Paschim Ramchandrapur to the sub-divisional health centre, the Namasudra in this location enjoy comparatively better medical facilities than the Namasudra of Kansona village, which is located at a far distance from sub-divisional health centre. The buttressed the rates of infant and toddler mortality among the study population residing in three different locations.

BIBLIOGRAPHY

Adak, D.K. (2001). A study of the phenomenon of demographic transition among the Ladiya of Madhya Pradesh. *Anthropologie*. XXXIX/2-2: 241-242.

____ (1993). *Mortality Pattern and its Biosocial Proximates: A Study on Tribal Populations of Shillong (Meghalaya)*. Ph.D. Thesis (unpublished). Guwahati University, Guwahati, Assam.

Adak, D.K. ; Sen Choudhury, S. and Choudhury, S. (1999). The Hajong of Meghalaya: A study on some demographic aspects. *Arunachal University Research Journal*, 2: 35-45.

Adak, D.K. and Gharami, A.K. (2001). A study on population composition of the Ladiya of Sagar district, Madhya Pradesh. *S.A. Antrhopol*. 1:83-89.

Adak, A and Suchindran, C.M. (1985). Factors affecting infant and child mortality. *J. Biosoc. Sci*. 17: 481 – 496.

Ali, S.G.M. (1968). Inbreeding and endogamy in Kerala. *Acta.Genet*. 18: 369-379.

Arora, G. (1990). *Social Structure and Fertility*. National Book Organisation, New Delhi.

Baker, P.T and Dutta, J.S. (1972). Demographic variables as measures of biological adaptation: A case study on high altitude human population. (In): G.A. Harrison and A.J. Boyee (eds.), *The Structure of Human Population*. Clarendon Press, Oxford, 352-378.

Baltzar, C.J. and Solon, S.F. (1989). Disposal of faeces of children under two years old and diarrhoea incidence, a case control study. *Int. J. Epidemiol*. 18: 516-519.

Bankole, A. (1994). *The Role of Mass Media in Family Planning Promotion in Nigeria*. DHS Working Papers No. 11 . Macro International, Calverton, Maryland.

Bardhan, A. (1966). *Relationship of Physique with Menarche of the Punjabi and Bengalee Girls*. Ph.D. Thesis (unpublished). University of Delhi, Delhi.

Basu, A. (1986). Genetics, socio-cultural and health care practices among tribal groups of Jagdalpur and Konta Teshsils of Bastar district, M.P. (In): A.K. Kalla and K.S. Singh (eds.), *Anthropology and Nation Building*. Concept Publishing Company, New Delhi, 87-105.

Basu, A.M. (1987). Household influences on childhood mortality : Evidence from historical and recent mortality trends. *Soc. Biol*. 34 : 187 – 205.

Basu, D; Guha, M and Dutta, U. (1992). Palmar dermatoglyphic profile of Bangladesh Namasudra immigrants in the Mana refugee camp Raipur, M.P. *Man in India*. 72 : 105-113.

Basu, S.K. (1971). Consanguinity in India. *Adivasis*. XII : 1- 4.

______ (1975). Effects of consanguinity among north Indian Muslims. *J. Pop. Res*. 2: 51-58.

______ (1978). Effects of consanguinity among Muslims group of India. In: I.C. Verma (ed.), *Medical Genetics in India*. Vol. 2. Auroma Enterprises, Pondichorry, 173-178.

______(1989). Factors effecting fertility and mortality behaviour among tribal groups of Bastar District, Madhya Pradesh. (In): B. Jena and R.N. Pati (eds.), *Health and Family Welfare Services in India*. Ashish Publishing House, New Delhi, 353-362.

Bean, R. and Wood, C. (1974). Ethnic variations in relationship between income and fertility. *Demography*. 11 : 629.

Bebarta, P.C. (1977). *Family type and Fertility in India*. Christopher, North Quincy.

Behraman, J.R. (1998). Intra Household Allocation of Resources : Is there a Gender Bias? (In) : *Too Young To Die* : Genes or Gender? United Nations, New York, 223-242.

Berman, P.; Kendall, C. and Bhattacharya, K. (1994). The household production of health : Integrating social science perspectives on micro-level health determinants. *Soc. Sci. Med.* 38: 205-215.

Berrai, J.; Cann, H.M.; Cavallik –Sfooza, L.L. and P. De. Hicola (1968). The effects of parental age on rates of maturation for haemophilia A and B. *Am. J. Hum. Genet*. 20 : 175-196.

Bertrand, J.T.; Santiso, R.; Linder, S.H. and Pinda, M.A. (1987). Evaluation of a communications programme to increase adoption of vasectomy in Guatemala. Stud. *Farm. Plann.* 16:361.

Bhanot, I.V. and Gandotra, M.M. (1970). Baroda fertility study – A brief report. (In): A. Bose; P.B. Desai and S.P. Jain (eds.), *Studies in Demography*. Allen and Unwin Ltd. London, 473-484.

Bharati, P. and Ghoshadastidar, M. (1990). Maternal education, fertility and mortality in a Bengali population sample. *J. Ind. Anthrop. Soc.* 25: 90-93.

Bhatia, J.C. and Cleland, J. (1995). Determinants of maternal care in region of South India. *Hlth. Trans. Rev*. 5: 127-142.

Biswas, N.C. (1967). Age of menarche among Punjabi girls of Delhi. *Anthropol*. 14:153-170.

Bogue, D.J. (1966). Family planning research :An outline of the field. In: Berelson *et al.* (eds.), *Family Planning and Population Programs*. University of Chicago Press, Chicago.

_______(1969). *Principles of Demography*. Wiley, New York.

Bolam, A.; Manandhar, D.S.; Shrestha, P.; Ellis, M. and Costello,

A.M. (1998). The effects of postnatal health education for mothers on infant care and family planning practices in Nepal : A randomized controlled trial. *Br. Med. J.* 316: 805-811.

Bose, N.K. (1975). *The Structure of Hindu Society*. Orient Longman Ltd., New Delhi.

Brebant, V. (1954). Tendences de la fecondite on Conge, Belge (In): *World Population Conference*. Document 349. United Nations, Rome.

Briscoe, J.; Baltazor, J. and Young, B. (1988). Case control studies of the effect of environmental sanitation on diarrhoea morbidity: Methodological implications of field studies in Africa and Asia, *Int. J. Epidemiol*. 17:441-447.

Brito, E. (1952). A poligamia e a natalidade entre OS grupos ethnicos Manjaco, Balanta e Brame. *Boletini Cultural de Guine Portuguesa*. 7: 161.

Buchanan, R. (1975). Breast feeding : Aid to infant health and fertility control. *Population Reports*. Series J. No. 4: 503-510.

Buck, C. and Stavarky, K. (1967). The relationship between age at menarch and age at marriage among child bearing women. *Hum. Biol*. 39: 53-64.

Bumpass, L. (1969). Age at marriage as a variable in socio-economic differential in fertility. *Demography*. 6: 45-54.

Busia, K.A. (1954). Some aspects of the relations of social conditions on human fertility in the Gold Coast. (In) : F. Lorimer (ed.), *Culture and Human Fertility*. UNESCO, Paris, 341.

Butz, W.R. and Davanzo, J. (1978). *Contracepting, breast feeding and birth spacing in Malaysia : A model of decision making subject to economic and biological constraints*. A preliminary paper. Rand Corporation, USA.

Butz, W.R.; Habicht, J.P. and Da Vanzo, J. (1984). Environmental factors in the relationship between breastfeeding and infant mortality. The role of sanitation and water in Malaysia. *Am. J. Epidemiol*. 119: 516.

Caldwell, J.C. (1979). Education as a factor of mortality decline : An examination of Nigerian data. *Popul. Stud.* 33: 395.

Caldwell, J.C.; Reddy, P.H. and Caldwell, P. (1996). The family in South India : Past, present and future. *Soc. Change.* 26: 116-129.

_______and ______ (1983). The social components of mortality decline : An investigation in south India employing alternative methodologies. *Popul. Stud.* 37: 185-205.

Census of India (1991). *West Bengal, Series 26, Vol. – A and B. Scheduled Castes and Scheduled Tribes.* Office of the Registrar General on India. Government of India, New Delhi.

Census of India (1971 and 1981). *West Bengal. Series 26, Vol. -- I and II. Scheduled Castes and Scheduled Tribes.* Office of the Registrar General of India. Government of India, New Delhi.

Census of India (1971). *Special Tables on Scheduled Castes and Scheduled Tribes West Bengal.* Series 22, Part 5(A), Controller of Publications, New Delhi.

Census of India (1981). *Final Population Tables, Total Population, Scheduled Castes Population and Scheduled Tribes Population, West Bengal.* Series 23. Directorate of Census Operation, Calcutta.

Census of India (1991). *Census of India, West Bengal, District Census Handbook. North 24 Paraganas* Series 26 Part XII-A. Directorate of Census Operations, West Bengal.

Chachra, S.P. and Bhasin, M.K. (1998). Anthropo – demographic study among the caste and tribal groups of central Himalayas: 1. Population Structure. *J. Hum. Ecol.* 9: 405-416.

Chakki, D.A. (1974). Modernisation and social change : The family and kin network in urban India. (In) : G. Kurian (ed.), Family in India : A Regional View. *Studies in the Social Sciences,* Vol-12. Mouton, Paris, 205-231.

Chakravorty, M.R. (1968). Consanguinity in India, *Z. Morph. Anthrop.* 60: 170-182.

Chakravorty, M.R. and Chakravorty, R. (1977). Genetic bearing of the sex ratio. *Ind. Anthrop.* 1: 56-71.

Chakravorty, R and Chakrvorty, R. (1973). *On consanguineous marriages and the genetic load.* II. Ann. Conf. Ind. Soc. Hum. Genet, Calcutta.

Chandna, R.C. (1999). *Population. Kalyani Popular Science.* Kalyani Publishers, New Delhi.

Chandra, R.K. (1978). Immunological aspects of human milk. *Nutr. Rev.* 36: 265.

Chandrasekhar, S. (1972). *Infant Mortality, Population Growth and Family Planning in India.* Allen and Unwin, London.

Chandrasekharan, N.C. (1959). Cultural factors and propagation of family planning in the Indian setting. *J. Fam. Welf.* 5: 43-51.

Chang, G.C.; Warren, R.D. and Pendleton, B.F. (1979). Testing and clarifying a macro model of socioeconomic change and fertility. *Soc. Biol.* 26:30.

Chatterjee, M. (1989). Competence and care for women : Health policy perspectives in the household context. (In) : M. Krishnaj and K. Chanana (eds.), *Gender and the Household Domain : Social and Cultural Dimensions. Women and the Household in Asia.* No. 4. Sage Publications, London, 165-190.

Chauhan, J.S. (1974). Age at marriage : A study of 400 mothers obtaining maternity services at a metropolitan teaching hospital. *J. Fam. Welf.* 20: 40-48.

Chowdhury, D.; Behera, M.C. and Adak, D.K. (1994). Some bio-demographic aspects of the khamti and its demographic transition. (In) : S. Mukherjee; F. I. Hussain; P. Chakraborty and G. Das. (eds.), *Demographic Profile of North East India*, Omsons Publications, New Delhi.

Clarke, L.L and Coward, R.T. (1991). A multivariate assessment of the effects of residence on infant mortality. *J. Rur. Hlth.* 7: 246-265.

Clegg, E.J and Harrison, G.A. (1971). Reproduction in human high altitude population. *Hormones.* 2:13-25.

Cleland, J.G and Sathar, Z.A. (1984). The effect of birth spacing on childhood mortality in Pakisthan, *Popul. Stud.* 38: 401-418.

Colson, E. (1958). *Marriage and the Family Among the Plateau Tonga of Northern Rhodesia.* Manchester University Press, Manchester.

Coombs, L.C. (1979). Underlying family size preferences and reproductive behaviour. *Stud. Family Plann.* 10 : 25-36.

Culright, P.; Belt. S. and Scanzoni, J. (1974). Gender frequencies, sex predomination and family size in United States. *Soc, Biol.* 21 : 242-248.

Culwick, A.T. and Culwick, G.M. (1939). A study of population in Ulanga, Tanganyika Territory. *Social. Rev.* 30: 365.

Cunningham, A.S. (1983). Morbidity in breasfed and artificially fed children. *J. Pediat.* 90: 126.

Da Vanzo, J.; (1984). A household survey of child mortality determinants in Malaysia. *Popul. Dev. Rev.* 10 (Suppl): 307-322.

Da Vanzo, J.; Butz, W.P. and Habicht, J.P. (1983). How biological and behavioral influences on mortality in Malasiya vary during the first year of life. *Popul. Stud.* 37: 381-402.

Dandekar, K. (1974). Fertility : Its control and future prospects. (In): A. Bose (ed.), *Population in India's Development.* Vikas Publishing House, New Delhi, 334-342.

______(1959). *Demographic Survey of Six Rural Communities.* Publication 37. Gokhale Institute of Politics and Economics, Poona, Bombay.

Dasgupta, M. (1987). Selective discriminations against female children in rural Punjab, India, *Popul. Dev. Rev.* 13: 77-100.

Davidson, M. (1970). Social and economic variations in child spacing. *Soc. Biol.* 17:107-113.

Davis, K and Blake, J. (1956). Social structure and fertility : An analytical framework. *Econ. Dev. Cult. Change.* 4:211.

De Sweemer, C. (1984). The influence of child spacing on child survival. *Popul. Stud.* 38: 47-72.

District Statistical Hand Book, North Twenty Four Parganas (1996 and 1997 combined). *Bureau of Applied Economics and Statistics*, Government of West Bengal, Calcutta.

Daon, R.M. and Bishart, L. (1990). Female autonomy and child nutritional status : The extended family residential unit in Amman, Jordan. *Soc. Sci. Med.* 31: 783-789.

Dorjahn, V.R. (1959). The factor of polygyny in African demography. (In) : W. Bascom and N. Herskovits (eds.), *Continuity and Change in African Culture*, University of Chicago Press, Chicago, 87.

Drejer, R. (1991). Childbirth at home can be both safe and emotionally fulfilling. *Wld. Hlth. Forum*. 12: 10-11.

Driver, E.D. (1963). *Differential Fertility in Central India*. Princeton University Press, Princeton.

____(1963). *Differential Fertility in India*. Princeton University Press, Princeton.

Dronamraju, K.R. and Meera Khan, K.C. (1963). A study of Andhra Pradesh : Consanguinity, caste literacy and bridal age. *Acta. Genet*. 13: 21-29.

Dutt, J.S. (1980). Altitude and fertility: The compounding effect of childhood mortality – A Bolivian example. *Soc. Biol*. 27: 101-113.

Dutta, N.K. (1986). *Origin and Growth of Caste in India* (Vol. – I and II). Farma, K.L. Mukhapadhya Pvt. Ltd, Calcutta.

Encyclopaedia Britanica (1983). William Benton Publisher, Chicago.

ESCAP (1988). Infant and Child Mortality : The Implications for Fertility Behaviour. *Population Research Leads*, No. 29. ESCAP, Bangkok.

Fawcett, J.T. and Bornstein, M.H. (1973). Modernization, individual modernity and fertility. (In): J.T. Fawcett (ed.), *Psychological Perspectives on Population. Basic Books*, New York, 106.

Foege, W.H. (1983). Prevention and care of prevalent infections in the mother and the newborn. (In) : F.D. Mundo et al. (eds.),

Primary Maternal and Neonatal Health. Plenum Press, New York.

Forste, R. (1994). The effects of breast feeding and birth spacing on infant and child mortality in Bolivia. *Popul. Stud.* 48: 497-511.

Freedman, R. (1963). Norms for family size in underdeveloped countries. In : M. Krishnaj and K. Chanana (eds.), *Population and Society*. Houghton Miffin, Boston, 215.

______(1967). Application of the behavioral sciences to family planning. *Stud. Fam. Plann.* 23: 5-9.

Freedman, R. and Coombs. L. (1966). Child spacing and family economic position. *Am. Social Review*. 31: 361-648.

Freedman, R.; Takeshita, J.Y. and Sun, T.H. (1964). Fertility and family planning in Taiwan : A case study of demographic transition. *Am. J. Social*. 70:16.

Frisancho, A.; Roberts, K.; Jane, E. and Matos, J. (1976). Symbolic relationship of high fertility, high childhood mortality and socio-economic status in an urban Peruvian population. *Hum. Biol.* 48: 101-111.

George, M. (1973). Tradition and fertility in a rural community. *Ind. J. Soc. Work*. 34:1.

Ghatak, N.K. (1990). Namasudra of Bengal through the Ages. *Bulletin of the Cultural Research Institute*. 17: 18-21.

Ghosh, S.L. (1978). *West Bengal*. National Book Trust, New Delhi.

Goldberg, H.I.; Rodrigues, W.; Thome, A.M.; Janowitz, B. and Morris, L. (1984). Infant mortality and brestfeeding in North-Eastern Brazil. *Popul. Stud.* 38: 105.

Golladay, T. (1980). *Health – Sector Policy* Paper. World Bank, Washington, D.C.

Goode, W.J. (1963). *World Revolution and Family Patterns*. Free Press of Glencoe, London.

Gore, M.S. (1965). The traditional Indian family. In: M.F. Nimkoff (ed.), *Comparative Family System*. Houghton Miffin, Boston, 209.

Goyal, R.P. (1974). Fertility and family planning in urban Delhi. (In) A. Bose et al. (eds.), *Population in India's Development* : 1947 – 2000. Vikash Publishing House, New Delhi.

______(1975). Shift in age at marriage in India between 1961-1971. *Demography India*. 4: 336-344.

Grabill, W.H.; Kiser, C.V. and Whelpton, P.K. (1958). *The Fertility of American Women*. Wiley, New York.

Grabill, W.H. and Davidson, M. (1968). Recent trends in child spacing among American Women. *Demography*. 5: 212-225.

Grant, J.P. (1994). *State of the World's Children*. UNICEF, Oxford.

Gubhaju, B.B.; Streatfield, K. and Mazumder, A.K. (1991). Socio-economic demographic and environmental determinants of infant mortality in Nepal. *J. Biosoc. Sci*. 23: 425-435.

Gabhajum, B.B. (1985). Effect of birth order and maternal age on infant and child mortality in rural Nepal. *Biol. Society*. 2: 15-22.

Gupta, R.P. (1998). Health facilities and health achievements in four more backward states of India M.P. *J. Soc. Sci*. 3: 44-63.

Gupta, R. Singh, K.L. and David, L.H. (1975). Fertility and fertility differentials in rural area. *J. Fam. Welf*. 21: 3-9.

Gustavus, S.O. and Nam, C.B. (1970). The formulation and stability of ideal family size among young people. *Demography*. 7: 43-51.

Hajnal, J. (1963). Age at marriage and proportions marrying. *Popul. Stud*. 7: 111.

Han, A.M. and Moe, K. (1990). Household faecal contamination and diarrhea risk.. *J. Trop. Med. Hyg*. 93: 333-336.

Henry, F.I. and Rahim, Z. (1990). Transmission of diarrhea in two crowded areas with different sanitary facilities in Dhaka, Bangladesh. *J. Trop. Med. Hyg*. 93: 121-126.

Henry, L. (1961). Some date on natural fertility. *Eugen. Qurt.* 8: 81.

Henry, L. (1976). *Population : Analysis and Methods*. Arnold, London.

Hill, R.S. (1959). *The family and Population Control – A Fuerto Rican Experiment in Social Change*. University of North Carolina Press, Chapel Hill.

Hobcrafi, J.; Mcdonald, J.W. and Rustein, S. (1985). Demographic determinants of infant and early child mortality : A comparative analysis. *Popul. Stud.* 39: 363-385.

______, ______, and ______(1983). Child spacing effects on infant and early child mortality. *Popul. Ind.* 49: 585-618.

Hotchkiss, D.R.; Nancy, B.M. and Seiber, E.E. (2002). The effect of the health care supply environment on children's nutritional status in rural Nepal. *J. Biosoc. Sci.* 34: 173-192.

Huttly, S.R.A.; Blum, D.; Kirkwood, B.R.; Emeh, R.N. and Feachem, R.G. (1987). The epidemiology of acute diarrhea in a rural community in Imo State, Nigeria. *Trans. Roy. Soc. Trop. Med. Hyg.* 81: 865-870.

Jain, A.K. (1985). Determinants of regional variation in infant mortality in rura! India. *Popul. Stud.* 39: 407-424.

Jain, A.K. and Bongaarts, J. (1981). Breastfeeding : Patterns, correlates and fertility effects. *Stud. Fam. Plann.* 12: 79-99.

James, W.H. (1969). Still birth, neonatal death and birth interval. *Ann. Hum Genet*. 32: 163-172.

Janowitz, B.; Lewis, J.H.; Parnell, A.; Hefnawi, F.; Younis, M.N. and Serour, G.A. (1981). Breastfeeding and child survival in Egypt. *J. Biosoc. Sci*. 13: 287-297.

Jelliffe, D.B. and Jelliffe, E.F.P. (1978). *Human Milk in the Modern World*. Oxford University Press, Oxford.

Khal, J.A. (1968). *The Measurement of Modernization, a Study of Values in Brazil and Mexico*. University of Taxas Press, Austin.

Karim, M.S. (1974). Fertility differentials by family type. Pakistan. *Dev. Rev.* 13:129.

Kelley, A. (1976). *Interaction of economic and demographic household behaviour. Paper presented at National Bureau of Economic Change in Less Developed Countries*, 1976. Philadelphia.

Khalifa, A. (1973). A proposed explanation of the fertility gap differentials by socio-economic status and modernity : The case of Egypt. *Popul Stud.* 27: 431.

_______(1976). The influence of wife's education on fertility in rural Egypt. *J. Biosoc. Sci.* 8: 53.

Khan, M.E. (1973). Factors affecting spacing of birth. *J. Fam. Welf.* 20: 54-67.

Khongsdhr, R. (1991). *A Bio-social, Demographic Study Among the War Khasi of Meghalaya*. M. Phil Dissertation (Unpublished). North Eastern Hill University, Shillong.

Knowles, J.C. and Anker, R. (1975). *Economic Determinants of Demographic Behaviour in Kenya. International Labour Review*. Population and Employment, Paper No. 28. The John Hopkins University Press, Baltimore.

Koenig, M.A.; Phillips, J.F.; Campbell, O.M. and D'souza, S. (1990). Birth intervals and childhood mortality in rural Bangladesh. *Demography*. 27: 251-265.

Kuate Defo, B. and Pilloni, A. (1995). Determinants of mortality among Cameroonian children : Are the effects of breast feeding and pace of childbearing artifacts ? *Genus. Sl.* (3-4) : 61-96.

Kumar, S., Pai and Swaminathan, M.S. (1967). Consanguineous marriages and the genetic load due to lethal gene in Kerala. *Ann. Hum. Genet.* 31: 141-147.

Lantz, P.; Partin, M. and Palloni, A. (1992). Using retrospective surveys for estimating the effects of breastfeeding and child spacing on infant and child mortality. *Popul. Stud.* 46: 121-139.

Lerner, D. (1958). *The Passing of Traditional Society*. Free Press of Glencoe, New York.

Lorimer, F. (1954). *Culture and Human Fertility*, UNESCO, Paris.

Lorimer, F.; Fortes, M.; Busia, K.A.; Richards, A.I.; Reining, P. and Mortara, G. (1954). *Culture and Human Fertility*. UNESCO, Paris.

Lowski, J. (1986). Mortality from acute respiratory infections in children under five years. *World Health Statstics*. Qurt. 39: 138-144.

Luella, K. (1974). Early teenage pregnancy contraception and repeat pregnancy. *Am. J. Obst. Gyn.* 120 : 249-256.

Mahadevan, K. (1979). *Sociology of Fertility: Determinants of Fertility Differentials in South India*. Sterling, New Delhi.

Mamdani, M. (1972). *The Myth of Population Control : Family, Caste and Class in an Indian Village,* Monthly Review Press, New York.

Manun, EBO. M.N.; Haggerty, P.A.; Kalengaie, M.; Ashworth, A. and Kirkwood, B.R. (1994). Influence of demographic, socio-economic and environmental variables on childhood diarrhea in a rural area of Zaire. *J. Trop. Med. Hyg*. 97: 31-35.

Marshal, J.F. (1972). A conceptual framework for viewing responses to family planning programs. *J. Cross Cultural Psychology*. 3: 1-21.

Mata, L.J and Wyatt. R.G. (1971). Host resistance to infection. *Am. J. Clin. Nutr*. 24: 976.

Matsunga, E. (1973). Effect of changing parental age patterns in chromosomal aberration and mutation. *Soc. Biol.* 20 : 82-88.

Matsunga, E and Tonomura, A. (1972). Parental age and birth weight in translocation Down's syndrome. *Ann. Hum. Genet*. 36: 209-219.

McCann. M.F.; Liskin, L.S.; Piotrow, P.T.; Rinehart, W. and Fox, G. (1981). *Breastfeeding, Fertility and Family Planning*. Population Report Series J. 24. Johns Hopkins University, Baltimore.

Meir, R. (1959). *Modern Science and Human Fertility Problem.* John Wiley and Sons. Inc., New York.

Memoria, C.B. (1965). *Population and Family Planning in India.* Kitab Mahal, Allahabad.

Merrick, T.W. (1985). The effect of piped water on early childhood mortality in urban Brazil, 1970-1976. *Demography.* 22: 1-24.

Milller, M.K.; Clarke, L.L.; Albrecht, S.L and Farmer, F.L. (1996). The interaction effects of race and ethnicity and mother's residence on the adequacy of parental care. *J. Rur. Hlth,* 12: 6-17.

Misra, B.D. (1982). *The Study of Population.* South Asian Publishers Pvt. Ltd,. New Delhi.

Mitra, A. (1978). *India's Population: Aspects of Quality and Control.* Vol – 1. Abhinav Publications, New Delhi.

Mitra, M. (2000). Health Culture and Health Seeking Behaviour among Abujhmaria and Kamar Primitive Tribes of Madhya Pradesh. (In) R. Chaubey and K.K.N. Sharma (eds.) *Tribal Health.* K.K. Publications, Allahabad.

Mitra, S. (1966). Income, socioeconomic status and fertility in the United States. *Eugen. Qurt.* 14: 223.

Mo-im, Kim. Rider; Rowland, V.; Harper, P.A. and Yang, Jae, Mo. (1974). Age at marriage, family planning practices and other variables as co-relates of fertility in Korea. *Demography.* 11 : 641-656.

Mubarak, S. (1989). Motherhood an end and a means. *Wld. Hlth. Forum.* 10: 247-248.

Muhsam, H.V. (1956). The fertility of polygynous marriage. *Popul. Stud.* 10: 3.

Muhuri, P.K. and Menken, J. (1997). Adverse effects of next birth, gender and family composition on child survival in rural Bangladesh. *Popul. Stud.* 51: 279-294.

Mukherjee, D.P. and Bhaskar, S. (1974). *Studies on inbreeding and its effect on same endogamous population of Chittoor District, Andhra Pradesh.* Ann. Conf. Ind. Soc.

Hum. Genet. Bombay.

Mukherjee, S.B. (1962). *Studies on Fertility Rates in Calcutta.* Bookland Pub, Calcutta.

Mukhopadhya, B. (1981). A comparative microdemographic study of two communities in coastal Midnapore district, West Bengal. *J. Biosoc. Sci.* 13, 479-489.

Murthy, P.S.N.; Ramnath, T.; Vijoyraghavan, K. and Rao, N.P. (1985). Nutritional profile of joint and nuclear families in rural Andhra Pradesh. *J. Fam, Welf.* 32: 80-87.

Mysore (1961). *The Mysore Population Study : A Co-operative Project of the United Nations and the Government of India.* Department of Economics and Social Affair, United Nations, New York.

Nag, M. (1962). *Factors Affecting Human Fertility in Non Industrial Societies : A Cross Cultural Study.* Department of Anthropology, Yale University, New Haven.

_______(1992). Sex preferences in Bangladesh, India and Pakistan and its effect on fertility. *Demography India.* 20 : 163-185.

Nair, P.M.; Anil Chandran, S. and Sabw. A. (2000). The effect of maternal health programmes on infant and child survival in India. *J. Fam. Welf.* 46: 61-63.

Nayar, P.K.B. (1974). The influence of education on fertility. *J. Fam. Welf.* 20: 28-35.

Novitsky, E. and Kimball, A.W. (1958). Birth order, parental ages and sex of offspring. *Am. J. Hum.* Genet. 10: 268-275.

Ohadike, P.O. (1968). A demographic note on marriage, family and family growth in Lagos, Nigeria, (In) : J.C. Caldwell and C. Okonjo (eds.), *The Population of Tropical Africa.* Columbia University Press, New York, 379.

Okore, A.O. (1977). *The Value of Children to Parents among the Ibos in Nigeria : A Case Study of Umuahia and Arochukwu in the East Central State.* Ph.D. Thesis. Department of Demography, Australian National University, Canberra.

Olusanya, P.O. (1971). The problem of multiple causation in population analysis with particular reference to the polygyny fertility hypothesis. *Soc. Rev.* 19: 165.

Opler, M.E. (1964). Cultural context and population control programs in village India. (In) : E.W. Count and G.T Bowles (eds.), *Fact and Theory of Social Science*. Syracuse University Press, Syracuse, 201.

Orenstein, H. (1966). The Hindu joint family : The norms and the members. *Pacific. Aff.* 39:314.

Orubuloye, I.O. (1977). *Fertility and Family Limitation in Nigeria: A comparative Study of Selected Rural Communities in Ekiti and Ibadan Division of the Western State*. Ph.D. Thesis. Department of Demography, Australion National University, Canberra.

Page, H.J. (1975). Fertility levels: Patterns and trends. (In): J.C. Caldwell (ed.), *Population Growth and Socioeconomic Change in West Africa*. Columbia University Press, New York.

Palloni, A. (1989). Effects of Inter-birth intervals on infant and early childhood mortality. (In) : L. Ruzicka; G. Wunsch and P. Kane (eds.), *Differential Mortality: Methodological Issues and Biosocial Factors*. Clarendon Press, Oxford, 163-188.

Palloni, A. and Millman, S. (1986). Effects of inter-birth intervals and breast feeding on infant and early childhood mortality. *Popul. Stud.* 40: 215-236.

Palmore, J.A. (1972). *Population change, conjugal status and the family. In : Population Aspects of Social Development*. Asian population studies Series No. II. ESCAP, Bangkok.

Pandey, G.D and Tiwary, R.S. (1993). Socio-cultural characteristics and health-seeking behaviour of the hill Korwas. *J. Fam. Welf.* 39:44.

Pandey, G.D; Verma, A and Tiwary, R.C. (1997). Some aspects of birth related practices in the Pondo tribe of Madhya Pradesh. *J. Fam. Welf.* 43 : 38-43.

Pandey, G.D. (2000). Differentials in Socio-Demographic Characteristics of Primitive Bharias of Madhya Pradesh. *Tribal Health Bulletin*, 6(3): 19-21.

Pandey, G.D. and Tiwary, R.S. (2000). A study on vital rates on the Primitive tribes of Madhya Pradesh. (In) R. Chaubey and K.K.N. Sharma (eds.), *Tribal Health*. K.K. Publications, Allahabad.

Pandey, G.D.; Verma, A. and Tiwary, R.S. (2001). Some correlates of infant mortality in a primitive tribe of Madhya Pradesh. *S.A. Anthropol*, I(I): 117-120.

Pandey, G.D. (2002). Maternal and Child Health care in Relation to Literacy in Bharias—A Primitive Tribe of Madhya Pradesh. (In) R. Chaubey and K. Saini (eds.), *Status of Women in Rural Societies*. Aditya Publishers, M.P.

Pant, P.D. (1996). *Infant and Child Mortality in Nepal : Social-economic, Demographic and Cultural Factors*. Ph.D. Thesis. Australian National University, Canberra.

Pareek, U and Kothandapani, V. (1969). Modernisation and attitudes to family size and family planning. *Soc. Biol*. 16: 44-48.

Patnaik, M.M. (1985). *Fertility Behaviour*. Janaki Publications, New Delhi.

Pearl, R. (1939). *The Natural History of Population*. Oxford University Press, Oxford.

Perez, A; Vela, P.; Masnick. G.S. and Polter, R.G. (1972). First ovulation after childbirth :The effect of breast feeding. *Am. J. Obs. Gyg*. 114: 1041-1047.

Piotrow, P.T.; Rimon, G.J.; Winnard, K.; Kincaid, D.L.; Huntington, D. and Conviser, J. (1990). Mass media family planning promotion in Nigeria Cities. *Stud. Fam. Plan*. 21: 265.

Plank, S.J. and Milanesi, M.L. (1973). Infant feeding and infant mortality in rural Chile. *WHO Bull*. 48: 203.

Pohlaman, E. (1969). *The Psychology of Birth Plannings*. Cambridge, Schenkman.

Poovan, P.; Kifle, F. and Kwast, B.E. (1990). A maternity waiting home reduces obsterics Catastrophes. *Wld. Hlth. Forum,* 11: 440-445.

Poston, D.L and Singlemann, J. (1975). Socioeconomic status, value orientations and fertility behaviour in India. *Demography*: 12:3.

Prakrasi, K. and Malaker, C. (1967). The relationship between family type and fertility. *Milbank Mem. Fund Qurt. Bull*. 45:451.

Rahman, M.; Rahman, M.M.; Wojtyniak, B. and Aziz, K.M.S. (1985). Impact of environmental sanitation and crowding on infant mortality in rural Bangladesh. *Lancet.* ii: 28-30.

Raina, B.L. (1969). *Family Size Norms in Population Problem in India*. Central Planning Institute, Bombay.

Rakshit, S. (1962). Reproductive life of same Maharastrian brahmin women . *Man in India*. 42: 139-149.

Rao, A.P. and Reddy, V. Rami (1977). Consanguineous marriages and their effects on fertility and offspring mortality in a rural Yadava population of South Eastern Andhra Pradesh. IV. Ann. Canf. *Ind. Soc. Hum.* Genet, Madras.

Rao, P.H. (1996). Family planning programme and contraceptive use in India: A marketing Perspective. *J. Fam. Welf.* 42: 21.

Rao, P.S.S and Inbaraj, S.G. (1979). Inbreeding effects on fertility and sterility in southern India, *J. Med. Genet*. 16: 24-31.

Rao, V.R. (1989). Population structure of Naik Gond of Chandrapur district, Maharashtra : A preliminary analysis. (In) : *Genetical Demography of India Population*. Anthropological Survey of India (ed.), Calcutta.

Reddy, Govinda. P. (1978). *Effects of consanguineous marriage on fertility and infant mortality among the Kappa and Mala of Southern Andhra Pradesh*. X. Int. Cong. Anthrop. Ethrol. Sci, India.

Reddy, K.N. (1991). *Population structure of Irulas of Nilgiris* (In) : K.N. Reddy and D.V. R. Rao (eds.), Population Structure among Tribes. Tamil University, Thanjavur. 1-138.

Reddy, V. Rami. (1977). *Age at menarche among the Balaji of*

Tirupati, south India. IV Ann. Genet. Cont., Madras.

Rele, J.R. (1963). Fertility differential in India. *Milbank Mem. Fund Quat*. 41:183-197.

______(1982). Trends and differentials in fertility. (In): *Population of India. Country Monograph Series*. No. 10. United Nations, New York.

Repetto, R. (1972). Son preference and fertility behaviour in developing countries. *Stud. Fam. Plan*. 3: 70-76.

Risley, H.H. (1891). *The Tribes and Castes of Bengal*. Bengal Secretariate Press. Vol.I: 183-189, Farma. K.L. Mukhapadhya Pvt. Ltd., Calcutta.

Robinson, M. (1951). Infant morbidity and mortality : A study of 3266 infants. *Lancet*. I:788.

Rosenstock, I.M. (1960). What research in motivation suggests for public health ? *Am. J. Pub. Health*. 50:295.

Ruzicka, L.T. and KANE, P. (1987). *Population Policies and Programmes: Current Status and Future Directions*. Asian Population Studies Series, No. 84. United Nations, New York.

Sadhu, K.K. (1987). *Bio-demographic Study of Kashmiris*. Gian Publishing House, New Delhi.

Saksena, D.N. (1973). *Differential Urban Fertility* Lucknow. Demographic Research Centre. Lucknow.

Sanghvi, L.D. (1966). Inbreeding in India : Inbreeding in the rural district of Andhra Pradesh. *Eugn. Quart*. 131: 291-293.

Sanghvi, L.D. (1978). The genetic consequences of inbreeding. (In). I.C. Verma (ed.), *Medical Genetics in India*. Auroma Enterprises, Pondicherry, 113-118.

Sarkar, N.C. (2000). Finger dermatoglyphics of the Namasudras of Nadia, West Bengal, India :Quantitative genetics. *J. Anthrop. Surv. India*. 49: 13-39.

Sechaiberg, A. (1970). Measuring modernism: Theoretical and empirical explorations. *Am. J. Soc*. 76: 399.

Seetha, M.V. (1957). Menarche and menopause in Andhra Pradesh. *J. Obs.Gyn. Ind*. 8: 79-82.

Selvin, S and Garfinkel, J. (1976). Parental age, maternal age and birth order and the risk of a foetal loss. *Hum. Biol.* 48 : 203-230.

Shah, A.M. (1973). *The Household Dimension of the Family in India*. Orient Longman, New Delhi.

Singh, I.P. (1999). Health seeking behaviour among the tribals of Rajasthan. (In): M.K. Bhasin and V. Bashim (eds.), *Rajasthan . Ecology, Culture and Society*. Kamala Raj Enterprises, New Delhi, 201-206.

Singh, K.P. (1989). *Corelates of Fertility Behaviour : A Study of Rural Communities in Punjab and Hariyana*. Concept Publication, New Delhi.

Smith, D.H. and Inkeles, A (1966). The OM Scale : A comparative socio-psychological measure of individual modernity. *Sociometry*. 29: 353.

Smith, J.E and Kunz, P.R. (1976). Polygyny and fertility in nineteenth century America. *Popul. Stud*. 39: 465.

Smith, T.E and Blacker, J.C.G. (1963). *Population Characteristics of the Commonwealth Countries of Tropical Africa*. Athlone Press, London.

Stanley, I. (1956). Notes on Mormon polygyny. West. Human. Rev. 10: 229.

Stanton, B.F.; Clemens, J.D. and Khair, T. (1988). Educational intervention for altering water-sanitation behaviour to reduce childhood diarrhea in urban Bangladesh : Impact on nutritional status. *Am. J. Clin. Nutr*. 48: 1162-1172.

Stinner, W.F and Madar, P.D. (1975). An analysis of family sex composition preference in the Philippines. *Demography*. 12: 67-69.

Stockwell, E.G. and Hutchinson, B.W. (1975). A note on mortality correlate of economic development. *Population Review*. 19: 46-50.

Stycos, J.M. (1958). Some directions for research on fertility control. *Milkbank. Meml. Fund. Qurt. Bull*. 36: 126.

Talwar, P.P. (1965). Adolescent sterility in an Indian population. *Hum. Biol*. 37: 256-261.

Thomas, I.M. (1987). Menarche and menopause in Tamil brahmins of India. *Man in India*. 67: 264-274.

Tinker, A. and Koblinsky, M.A. (1993). *Making Motherhood Safe*. Discussion Paper. The World Bank, Washington.

Tiwari, M.K.; Chakraborty, R.; Gupta, A. and D.K. Adak. (2002). The Raj Gond of Sagar District, M.P. : *A Demographic Study* (In press).

Trussell, J. and Hammerslough, C. (1983). A hazards model analysis of the covariates of infant and child mortality in Srilanka. *Demography*. 20: 1-26.

United Nations (1973). *The Determinats and Consequences of Population Trends*, Vol. 1 Population Studies, No. 50. United Nations, New York.

United Nations (1994). *Population and Development : Program of Action adopted at the International Conference on Population and Development*, September 5-13, Cairo.

United Nations (1998). *Mortality of Children Under Age 5 : World Estimates and Projections* (1950 – 2025). Population Studies No 105, United Nations, New York.

US Bureau of The Census (1953). *Current Population Report*. Series No. 46. Washington, D.C.

US Bureau of The Census (1950). *Current Population. Report*. Series No. – 27, Washington, D.C.

Van. DE Walle, E. (1968). Marriage in African censuses and inquiries (In): W. Brass (ed.), *Demography of Tropical Africa*. Princeton University Press, Princeton, 183.

Vanlandingham, M.; Trussell, J. and Grummerstrawn, L. (1991). Contraceptive and health benefits of breastfeeding : Areview of the recent evidence. *Int. Fam. Plann. Perspect*. 17: 131-136.

Vashisht, B.K. and Rana, R.K. (1991). Education, fertility and work participation of women. (In) : V.S. Mahajan (ed.), *Women's Contribution to India's Economic and Social Development*. Deep and Deep Publication, New Delhi, 345-347.

Victoria, C.G.; Smith, P.F.; Vaughan, J.P. and Nobre, L.C. (1988). Water supply sanitation and housing in relation to the risk of infant mortality from diarrhea. *Int. J. Epidemiol.* 17: 651-654.

Vlassoff, M. (1978). *Economic Motives and Fertility in an Indian Village*, Ph.D. Thesis (unpublished), University of Poona, India.

Walker, D. (2000). *The Untouchable Counter Elites of West Bengal*. D.L.B. Thakur, Harichand Mission, Kolkata.

Wailace, H.M. (1992). Maternal health antecedents of infant and early childhood mortality and morbidity. *J. Trop. Paediatr.* 38: 4-6.

Westoff, C.F. and Rodriguez, G. (1993). *The Mass Media and Family Planning in Kenya. DHS Working Papers* No. 4. Macro International Columbia, Maryland.

Whelpton, P.K. and Kiser, C.V. (Eds.) (1950). *Social and Psychological Factors Affecting Fertility*. Vol. II. Milbank Memorial Fund, New York.

Williamson, J. (1970). Subjective efficacy and ideal family size as predicators of favourability towards birth control. *Demography*. 7: 329.

World Health Organisation (1996) *Perinatal Mortality : A Listing of Available Information*. World Health Organisation, Geneva.

Wyon, John B. and Gordon, John E. (1971). The Khanna Study : *Population Problems in the Rural Punjab*. Harvard University Press, Cambridge.

Index

A

Adak, DK, 125, 126, 127

Age and sex structure, 41

Alma-Ata, 5

Anganwari workers, 38

Antenatal checkup, 108

Arora, Gomti, 8

Average live births, 76

B

Bandyapadhya, 19

Bardhan, 6

Basu, 9

Belief, 101

Bertrand, 11

Bhasin, 41

Bibhulibhusan, 8

Binod Bihari Biswas, 103

Blake, 6

Bongaon,
  block, 17
  literacy, 19
  susdivision, history, 17

Breast-feeding, 7, 11
  duration, 116

Briscoe, 7

Buchanan, 8

C

Caldwell, 9, 10

Chachra, 41

Chandals, 22

Chandna, 2

Chandrasekhar, 10

Child,
  age of, 116
  immunisation of, 118
  treatment of, 116

Clive, Lord, 16

Community Development Blocks, 130

Contraception, 121

D

Dandekar, 7, 11

Davis, 8

Delivery,
  attendant, 113
  place of, 111

Demographic characteristies, 41-72

Diarrhoea, 7

Diseases,
  treatment of, 101

Durga Biswas, 102

E

Educational status, 72

Encyclopaedia Britannica, 3

ESCAP, 2

Expected respondents, 110

F

Family planning,
  and fertility, 123
  method, 119

Fawcett, 10, 11

Fertility, 9

Fertility and infant mortality,
  and age at marriage, 93
  and economic status, 93
  and mother's education, 93
  and size of family, 93
  and type of family, 93

G

Gharami, 125

Ghatak, 13

Grabil, 10

Grant, 7

Gupta, 4, 8

H

Health, 3, 9, 10
  concept of, 101
  care, 5, 106
  care practices, 101-123
  care services, 37

Henry, 7

Huttly, 7

I

ICPD, 12

Immunisation, 4, 110

India, 2

Iron and folic acid tablets, 108

K

Kalipada Biswas, 103

Kansona, 30, 77, 87

Kane, 3

Kashyapa, 24

Khamti, 125

Khongsdier, 125

L

Land, 1

Larner, 10

Lorimer, 6

M

Madhya Pradesh, 7

Mahadevan, 7

Manu, 21

Mastunga, 7

Mirzafar, 16

Monogramy, 24

Mysore Population Study, 11

N

Nair, 108

Namasudra, 5, 21, 22
  death and funeral, 25
  diseases among, 104
  dress, 23
  family, 24
  food and drinks, 23
  gotra, 24
  habitation, 23
  inheritance and succession, 25
  marriage, 24
  occupation, 23
  religion, 25
  social structure, 24

Netai Biswas, 103

North Twenty-Four Parganas
  District, 15
  brief history, 16

Nutrition, 9

O

Occupational status, 72
  Ojha, 102

Okore, 6

Olusanya, 6

P

Pant, 12

Paschim Ramchandrapur, 30

Perez, 8

Pooran, 12

Population growth, 8

Pregnancy wastage, 89

Present study,
  discussion and conclusion, 124-133
  introduction, 1-13
  materials and methods, 36-40
  objectives, 13
  reviews of literature, 5

Purana Bongaon, 27

R

Raj Gonds, 126

Reddy, 41

Rele, 73

Reproductive
  behaviour, 2, 3
  performance, 73-100

Respondents,
  age of, 107
  education of, 108
  treatment of after delivery, 113

S

Sadhu, 6

Sarkar, 13

Sex ratio, 48

Shyamali Biswas, 103

Stockwell, 126

T

Talwar, 8

Tinker, 12

Tiwari, 127

U

UNICEF, 5

United Nations, 12

V

Van-de Walle, 6

Vashisht, 8

Victoria, 7

W

Wallace, 12

West Bengal, 1, 13, 14, 126, 130

Wise, Dr., 21

WHO, 3, 5

Wyon, 13

Y

Yanakura, 10